BASIC HEALTH PUBLICATIONS USER'S GUIDE

TO SPORTS NUTRIENTS

Learn What You Need to Know about Building Your Strength, Stamina, and Muscles.

DAVE TUTTLE

JACK CHALLEM Series Editor

The information contained in this book is based upon the research and personal and professional experiences of the author. It is not intended as a substitute for consulting with your physician or other healthcare provider. Any attempt to diagnose and treat an illness should be done under the direction of a healthcare professional.

The publisher does not advocate the use of any particular healthcare protocol but believes the information in this book should be available to the public. The publisher and author are not responsible for any adverse effects or consequences resulting from the use of the suggestions, preparations, or procedures discussed in this book. Should the reader have any questions concerning the appropriateness of any procedures or preparation mentioned, the author and the publisher strongly suggest consulting a professional healthcare advisor.

Series Editor: Jack Challem
Editor: Carol Rosenberg
Typesetter: Gary A. Rosenberg
Series Cover Designer: Mike Stromberg

Basic Health Publications User's Guides are published by Basic Health Publications, Inc.

ISBN: 978-1-59120-020-8 (Pbk.)
ISBN: 978-1-68162-874-5 (Hardcover)

CONTENTS

Introduction, 1

1. Protein Supplements and
   Meal-Replacement Powders, 3

2. Creatine, 11

3. Glutamine and Other Secretagogues, 23

4. Vitamins and Minerals, 31

5. Ecdysterone, 37

6. Ginseng and Astragalus, 42

7. Phosphatidylserine, 51

8. Methoxyisoflavone and Ipriflavone, 55

9. Ribose, 59

10. MSM, 63

11. Caffeine, Ephedrine, and Other
    Diet Aids, 67

12. Sports Drinks, 80

Conclusion, 85

Selected References, 86

Other Books and Resources, 88

Index, 90

INTRODUCTION

During the past decade, there has been an explosion of new sports-nutrition products. From meal-replacement powders to esoteric nutrients like ecdysterone and methoxyisoflavone, supplement companies are offering an unprecedented number of products that can build muscle, reduce recovery time, and enhance sports performance.

This has been a double-edged sword for consumers. On one hand, some of these new offerings are among the most powerful and effective nutrients ever sold. On the other hand, the vast numbers of available products can be confusing for even the most advanced athlete. Which products are the real winners, and which are also-rans? Since money doesn't grow on trees, how can you make the best choices for your particular sports needs and budget? This *User's Guide to Sports Nutrients* will answer these questions.

Some of the nutrients discussed in this book are probably familiar to you, such as protein powders and creatine. But do you know the best times to take these nutrients, and which of the available forms works best? By the time you finish this guide, you will have a comprehensive knowledge of these supplements, allowing you to use them to peak advantage in advancing your sports progress.

Other products are so new that you may not have heard about them yet. With fancy names like ipriflavone and phosphatidylserine, these complex molecules certainly sound like they should work. And many of them do. This guide will reveal the current state of research into these new kids on the block. Some have impressive bodies of scientific investigation behind them, while others have only animal studies to support their use. *User's Guide to Sports Nutrients* will tell it like it is, helping you to make decisions regarding your own purchases in this ever-changing field. This will include information on dosages, the need for on and off cycles to maintain effectiveness, and much more.

Everyone wants to get the biggest bang for their supplement bucks. You may have been disappointed that certain products didn't live up to their advertisers' claims, and as a result, you may be hesitant to sample new products. But you can't progress in your sports endeavors without trying new things. *User's Guide to Sports Nutrients* will provide you with the unbiased information you need to make the right choices.

CHAPTER 1

PROTEIN SUPPLEMENTS AND MEAL-REPLACEMENT POWDERS

It is hard to overemphasize the importance of protein in an athlete's diet. While there are numerous supplements that enhance protein synthesis, you can't synthesize new muscle proteins without adequate raw material—the amino acids in dietary protein. Training at a high intensity and then depriving your body of the protein it needs is like hitting your head against a wall. Nothing beneficial will result, and you could damage your hard-earned muscle growth in the process.

While it is theoretically possible to eat enough meat, fish, poultry, and dairy products to get the protein you need, most athletes find it difficult to do so. It takes time to fix meals and even more time to eat them and clean the dishes. This has led many busy men and women to get part of their protein requirements from protein powders and meal-replacement powders (MRPs).

Essential Building Blocks

Protein is an essential nutrient for all people, but especially for athletes. There is some protein in every single cell of the human body. Brain cells, for example, are 10 percent protein while red blood cells and muscle cells contain as much as 20 percent protein. All in all, protein makes up nearly 15 percent of your body weight, more than any other substance except water.

These body proteins have a wide range of functions, including tissue growth and development. Two protein-based filaments inside the muscle fiber, known as actin and myosin, are responsible for all muscle contraction. Tendons, ligaments, hair, skin, and nails are specialized kinds of structural proteins. Proteins are even needed to form most hormones, including insulin and growth hormone. The body manufactures all of these different proteins from amino acids.

Amino Acid
A component of dietary protein that contains nitrogen and other elements. The human body requires twenty amino acids to function properly.

The adult body can normally produce twelve of these amino acids on its own, hence the term "nonessential" amino acids. They are alanine, arginine, asparagine, aspartic acid, cysteine, glutamine, glutamic acid, glycine, histidine, proline, serine, and tryptophan. The other eight amino acids are called "essential" because they must be supplied by the diet. They are isoleucine, leucine, and valine (the branched-chain amino acids) plus lysine, methionine, phenylalanine, threonine, and tryptophan.

When your body has enough amino acids, you have a positive nitrogen balance. This means that you have sufficient nitrogen to support all of your body's needs with enough left over to permit muscle growth. Inadequate protein consumption relative to your needs results in a negative nitrogen balance.

Your Daily Protein Requirement

One of the main questions that athletes ask is how much protein they should consume. The U.S. Government has established a recommended intake of 0.8 grams per kilogram (g/kg) of body weight per day. That's equal to 0.36 grams per pound (g/lb). While some nutritionists maintain that this is a liberal allowance that provides enough protein for active individuals, recent research shows otherwise.

A number of studies, including several by Dr. Peter Lemon of the University of Western Ontario, show that most strength athletes need 1.7–1.8 g/kg (about 0.8 g/lb). Endurance athletes need a bit less: 1.2–1.4 g/kg (about 0.6 g/lb). These figures are based on total body weight. (Although body fat does not require protein, it is easier for athletes to compute their protein needs based on total body weight.)

Kilogram
Part of the metric system of measurement. A kilogram is equal to 1,000 grams and 2.2 pounds.

The foregoing requirements are for athletes who train three to four times per week. If you exercise more than this or train at a very high level of intensity, your protein requirement could be as high as 2.5 g/kg (1.1 g/lb) according to some researchers. For simplicity, try to maintain a daily intake of 1 g of protein per pound of body weight.

You need to eat an adequate amount of protein every day, even on the days you don't exercise. The body uses protein continuously to provide the raw materials for muscle growth, repair, and maintenance. However, only so much protein can be stored inside the muscle cells and in the blood and organs. So, if you consume too much protein at once, your body may eventually convert the excess into carbohydrate or fat.

At the same time, there is no scientific evidence to support the frequently heard idea that the body can assimilate only 35 g of protein at once. You can eat more than this amount per meal if you like, but it's better to spread out your protein consumption over three or four small meals to maintain relatively constant amino-acid levels throughout the day.

You can wind up with a negative nitrogen balance even at these recommended protein levels if you do not also consume enough carbohydrates. This can occur during the carbohydrate-depletion diets that are sometimes used prior to competitions with weight classes. It often occurs during long-distance marathon racing, too, as long-distance running dramatically depletes the body of carbohydrates.

When your body needs energy and does not have sufficient carbohydrates to meet its needs, it converts the protein in the liver and in the muscles into energy. This can result in a loss in muscle mass, as the body literally eats away at itself to get the nutrients it needs. Hardly what an athlete wants!

Protein Powders to the Rescue

It can be difficult to get enough protein from whole foods. Fortunately, a wide variety of protein supplements is now available. Soy, milk and egg, and whey powders each have their own special advantages. They also come in a wide variety of flavors to keep things interesting.

Soy powders are usually made from soy isolate, which is 99 percent protein. Because it is a vegetable protein, soy is low in methionine, although it is higher in glutamine than whey. Soy is also high in branched-chain amino acids and arginine, each of which is important for muscle growth. However, some of the plant chemicals in soy exert a mild estrogenic effect, which can reduce muscle definition, so male athletes should not consume large amounts of soy.

Milk and egg powders are protein blends. Originally made from powdered milk, they now contain a variety of milk components. As cheese is produced, the milk divides into two main products: a solid portion called *casein* and a liquid known as *whey*. Milk and egg powders combine various amounts of these fractions, usually adding some egg white (also called albumin) to the mix.

Scientists have learned that casein and whey have their own unique characteristics. Casein is assimilated relatively slowly, so it provides a steadier flow of amino acids to the bloodstream. This allows it to significantly reduce protein breakdown. Casein also has larger amounts of the amino acids that can be used for energy during exercise. However, because casein contains lactose, it can cause gastrointestinal distress in individuals who lack the enzyme lactase, which breaks down lactose. Whey, on the other hand, is assimilated very quickly, so it boosts protein synthesis much more than casein.

Whey: The Market Leader

Most of the protein powders on the market today are whey powders. In the early nineties, scientists developed a number of systems, including ion-exchange and microfiltration, to distill whey into a high-quality product that is nearly fat- and lactose-free. These systems use cool temperatures that preserve the taste and natural configurations of the amino acids.

Whey has the highest bioavailability of any protein. It dissolves easily in water, allowing the athlete to mix a protein drink on the run. While whey has less glutamine, arginine, and phenylalanine than either casein or soy, its ability to dramatically increase protein synthesis has made it a favorite of athletes. Whey also has immune-enhancing properties due to its ability to increase levels of the antioxidant glutathione.

Bioavailability
A measure of how much of an orally consumed nutrient actually passes through the intestinal tract wall so it can be utilized by the body.

Whey isolate is the purest form of whey. It has less moisture and lactose than whey concentrate, so gram for gram you get more protein for your money than with whey concentrate. However, whey isolate costs more than whey concentrate, so there is a trade-off. Whey products that use the old high-temperature process cost less but are not as effective because the proteins are denatured and less biologically active.

Remember that these supplements are not intended to replace the protein in your regular meals. Their value lies in giving you an easy way to get additional protein when your meals do not provide enough to meet your daily requirement.

They can therefore help you to achieve the goals you have set for your sport.

Meal Replacements Offer Convenient Nutrition

Numerous studies have shown that the best way to build muscle and lose fat at the same time is to eat five or six small meals spread throughout the day. Such a division of food intake provides a steady stream of protein, promoting maximum growth. Each meal has a thermic effect as well, which boosts your metabolic rate and minimizes the amount that is stored as fat. Moreover, dividing your carb intake into smaller portions helps to restore your muscle glycogen without fat accumulation.

Glycogen
The storage form of glucose (blood sugar). Found primarily in the liver and muscle fibers, it is one-third glucose and two-thirds water.

But who has the time and energy to prepare and eat five or six meals from whole foods each day? Not most athletes, to be sure. With their work, training, family, and other obligations, athletes need a convenient way to get nourishment on the run, and meal-replacement powders (MRPs) provide the answer to their needs.

These powders are usually high in protein, moderately high in carbohydrates, and low in fat. Most can be mixed with water in a shaker to form a flavorful drink, although some need to be prepared with a blender. Several of them become very thick (due to the guar gum and other thickeners that they contain), while others have the consistency of chocolate milk. They are artificially sweetened and therefore have a low sugar content, even when they contain substantial amounts of carbs.

Many Different Ingredients

A survey of the MRPs currently on the market shows that the protein content ranges from 25–52 g per serving with anywhere from 9–28 g of carbs. Fat content is always very low—no more than 4.5 g. Based on the total number of calories per single-serving packet, the macronutrient ratio of these MRPs ranges from 52 to 73 percent protein, from 19 to 41 percent carbohydrate, and from 0 to 14 percent fat. Total caloric value varies from 170–340 calories per serving.

The main protein in most MRPs is whey—usually whey concentrate but sometimes a blend of whey isolate, concentrate, and hydrolysate. Some products combine whey with casein and egg albumin to provide a more slowly assimilated blend of amino acids. A number of products also include protein-based growth factors and bioactive peptides, such as casomorphins, immunoglobulins, glycomacropeptides, IGF-1, and lactoferrin, which help to promote muscle growth and repair while providing support for your immune system.

The carbohydrate content usually comes from maltodextrin, brown-rice complex, fructooligosaccharides, fructose, corn-syrup solids, and/or sucrose. Fat sources consist of medium-chain triglycerides, borage oil, flaxseed oil, coconut oil, sunflower oil, and/or sometimes partially hydrogenated oils.

Many manufacturers also add a variety of sports-related nutrients to their formulations. Some of the more common nutrients are chromium, glutamine, taurine, tyrosine, creatine monohydrate, branched-chain amino acids, hydroxymethylbutyrate (HMB), and alpha-ketoglutarate. Fat burners and blockers are occasionally included as well, such as hydroxy-citric acid (HCA), lecithin, choline, inositol, carnitine, and chitosan. MRPs are also fortified with vitamins and minerals, ranging from 33 to 100 percent of the recommended daily value per serving.

There are many flavors available, so there is no reason to get bored with your MRP. In addition to the standard chocolate, vanilla, and strawberry, the selection includes orange, wild berry, chocolate peanut butter, and even a variety pack of tropical flavors.

Picking the Best Product for You

With so much diversity, you need to carefully select the product that is right for you. Figure out your total daily protein requirement and subtract the amount you obtain from whole-food sources. The remainder is what you need to get from a protein supplement or MRP.

As far as carbs are concerned, your daily requirement depends on your metabolism and energy expenditure. Most athletes require 2–3 g of carbs per pound of body weight. Do the math and determine how many carbs you need each day. Then divide the total between MRPs and dietary carbs such as oatmeal, whole-grain breads, pasta, legumes, and potatoes.

Even if you are extremely busy, you should try to get at least half of your carb intake from whole food. While the carbs in MRPs tend to be fairly low on the glycemic index, they contain virtually no fiber—an important part of a balanced diet. The fat content of MRPs and protein powders is so low that it should not impact your waistline.

When used appropriately, these powders can help you to achieve your sports objectives. They provide the nutrients you need for muscle growth without excessive calories, allowing you to control your body-fat level as you pursue peak performance. MRPs and protein powders are tailor-made for the fast-paced, active lifestyle of athletes, so be sure to include them in your dietary regimen.

CHAPTER 2

CREATINE

Of all the sports supplements available, none has been more extensively studied than creatine. This white, odorless powder burst onto the sports scene in the mid-nineties and transformed the supplement industry in the process. Initially, only creatine monohydrate was available, but soon creatine citrate followed, along with effervescent creatine, liquid creatine, creatine-transport drinks, and even creatine candy.

It has been nearly a decade since creatine first appeared, which means it has outlasted the usual two- or three-year window for a supplement fad. Why? Because creatine works for most everyone in a wide variety of sports. It increases energy and strength, which translates into more muscle mass and greater performance for athletes—particularly those in sports that involve short bursts of maximal intensity.

Your Three Energy Pathways

Creatine is an essential player in one of the three primary energy systems used for muscle contraction. It exists in two different forms within the muscle fiber: as free (chemically unbound) creatine and as creatine phosphate (CP). This latter form of creatine makes up two-thirds of your total creatine supply.

ATP
The "energy currency" for your cells. ATP is composed of one adenosine molecule and three phosphate molecules.

When your muscles contract, the initial fuel for this movement is a compound called adenosine triphosphate (ATP).

ATP releases one of its phosphate molecules to provide energy for muscle contraction and other functions. Once ATP releases a phosphate molecule, it becomes a different compound called ADP (adenosine diphosphate). Unfortunately, there is only enough ATP to provide energy for about ten seconds, so for this energy system to continue, more ATP must be produced.

Creatine phosphate (CP) comes to the rescue by giving up its phosphate molecule to ADP, recreating ATP. This ATP can then be "burned" again as fuel for more muscle contraction. The bottom line is that your ability to regenerate ATP largely depends on your supply of creatine. The more creatine you have in your muscles, the more ATP you can remake.

This greater ATP resynthesis keeps your body from relying as much on another energy pathway called glycolysis, which has lactic acid as a byproduct. This acid irritates the muscle fiber, causing pain. Eventually lactic-acid levels rise so high that they interfere with the biochemical reactions needed for muscle contraction. So, if you have less lactic acid in your muscles, you can train longer and gain strength, power, and muscle size. You also don't get tired as quickly.

In less than a minute, your demands for energy exceed the limits of the ATP-CP pathway, and you start to produce energy through glycolysis. If you train long enough at a high enough intensity, you will get so much lactic acid in your muscles that you will have to temporarily stop working out. Anyone who has given his or her all in the gym or on the playing field knows this feeling.

The third energy pathway is the aerobic pathway. It can be utilized only when adequate oxygen is available. This occurs when the sports activity involves less than maximal effort, even though you can get tired if you do enough of it. Submaximal activities, such as jogging, treadmill walking, and of course "aerobics" classes primarily use this energy pathway, which does not involve creatine.

A Natural Nutrient

Creatine is naturally present in your body at a level of around 0.75 g per pound of body weight. Approximately 95 percent of the total supply is found in the skeletal muscles. The remaining 5 percent is scattered throughout the rest of the body, with the highest concentrations in the heart, brain, and testes. (Sperm is chock-full of creatine!)

The body gets its creatine from two sources: food and its own internal production. Creatine is found in moderate amounts in most meats and fish, which are, after all, skeletal muscles. Good sources of dietary creatine include beef, chicken, turkey, tuna, cod, salmon, and pork. Tiny amounts are found in milk and even cranberries. Unfortunately, cooking destroys part of the creatine that exists in these foods.

The body can also make creatine using the three amino acids arginine, glycine, and methionine as raw material. This production occurs in the liver, pancreas, and kidneys. The body will manufacture only so much on its own, however. If you want to maximize the creatine stores in your muscles, you need to take a creatine supplement.

Please note that the creatine on store shelves is synthesized in a factory from chemicals. No one grinds up meat to get creatine. This manufacturing process can produce modest amounts of impurities if the factory owner is not careful. (The Chinese creatine available a few years ago was notorious for its impurity levels.)

To make sure that you get minimal impurities in your creatine monohydrate, use a brand that says "Creapure" on the label. These brands are made with a patented technology. Creatine is very affordable nowadays, so it is silly to put impurities in your body just to save a couple of bucks.

Mountains of Research

Unlike some supplements that have only rat or test-tube studies to support their use, creatine has been the subject of hundreds of published clinical trials. Most of these studies involved athletes, giving us an unprecedented level of certainty about creatine's benefits.

There has been so much research on creatine that you could write a book about it. In fact, I did—with Ray Sahelian, M.D., called *Creatine: Nature's Muscle Builder* (Avery Publishing, 1999). Check out this book if you want to learn the many details of this exciting supplement.

Virtually all of the available research has been done with creatine monohydrate, a powder with a neutral taste that is stable until put in water. Creatine monohydrate in moderate amounts is easily absorbed in the intestinal tract and raises blood levels of creatine within an hour.

Once in the muscle cell, creatine remains there for up to a month. Creatine can occasionally be converted in the body to creatinine, a harmless but useless substance that is filtered by the kidneys and excreted in urine. Creatinine is also produced when creatine remains in water for extended periods.

Not everyone benefits from creatine supplementation. One study found that up to 30 percent of users are nonresponders. It is not known why this occurs, but it is thought to relate to the amount of creatine you store naturally. While the average concentration in muscle tissue is 125 mmol (millimoles per liter), normal creatine levels can range from 100–160 mmol. If your muscles are already at or near this maximum concentration, you may not experience an increase in strength or sports performance. The only way to tell is to try creatine and find out for yourself.

The Athletes Who Benefit Most

Because creatine is involved in the energy pathway

used for bursts of explosive power, it should not be surprising that athletes in sports relying heavily on this pathway derive the greatest benefits. This includes bodybuilders, powerlifters, wrestlers, short-distance track and field athletes, and football and hockey players.

Studies at the Karolinska Institute in Sweden found that a dose of 20 g of creatine monohydrate per day produced an average 5 percent increase in peak torque (a measure of force production) and similar gains in the amount of work performed. The subjects also gained an average of 2.4 pounds of body weight during the one-month experiment.

A study at three Texan research institutions found significant increases in strength from creatine mono-hydrate. The male volunteers, who regularly trained with weights, got stronger and more muscular from a regimen of 20 g of creatine per day for twenty-eight days. After four weeks, the amount of weight they could lift for one repetition (1-RM) rose by 8.2 kg (more than eighteen pounds), and the number of reps they could do at 70 percent 1-RM rose from eleven to fifteen. They also gained an average of 3.7 pounds of body weight with only a 0.2 pound increase in body fat. That means that 95 percent of the gain was muscle mass!

So many studies have been performed with athletes that it is impossible to list them all in this short book. Suffice it to say that any athlete who relies strictly on strength and power will benefit from creatine use. The only times when creatine is not recommended is when other factors influence performance, such as body weight.

For a bodybuilder, more weight is great—as long as it's lean muscle. Ditto for wrestlers, power-lifters, and other strength athletes. But if you are a marathon runner, the increased body weight may slow you down, even if you are stronger. For this reason, marathon runners and triathletes should sample creatine in the off-season to see what trade-offs they experience. The increased muscle mass could also prove counterproductive for swimmers and martial artists, although the greater power and speed would be beneficial. Again, an off-season trial is recommended.

Creatine Monohydrate versus Creatine Citrate

Creatine monohydrate is a molecule of creatine attached to one molecule of water (*mono* means "one"), while creatine citrate has a molecule of creatine and a molecule of citrate. The creatine is identical in both cases, but the carrier molecule changes the total package somewhat.

Gram for gram, creatine monohydrate has more creatine than creatine citrate. Creatine monohydrate is about 60 percent creatine, while creatine citrate is only 40 percent creatine. This means you need to take a bit more creatine citrate to get the same effects, so be sure to look at the label to see what creatine you are getting.

While no published research has compared the performance benefits of monohydrate with citrate directly, an Italian study found that the absorption rates of both forms are about the same. Also, please note that some manufacturers list the amount of creatine in the product instead of the total with the carrier molecule attached, so check the label. You may be getting more creatine than you thought at first glance.

One supposed advantage of creatine citrate is that it does not cause "bloating." The argument is that your body takes in added water with creatine monohydrate, which can boost the amount of water in your skin. But even if the hydrate molecule is assimilated, the amount you consume is unlikely to cause noticeable bloating.

A 5-g dose of creatine monohydrate has 2 g of water, so you would be taking in one ounce (28 g) of water every two weeks. That's peanuts compared with the amount you drink. Also, there is virtually no creatine in the skin, so the bloating would not occur there. Rather, it would take place inside your muscle cells—precisely where you want it.

It is true that creatine monohydrate increases water levels inside the muscle cell. This is one of the reasons why it works, because higher intramuscular water levels boost protein synthesis and muscle growth. Since creatine citrate is effective, it probably does the same thing. However, there is so little research on creatine citrate that much remains unknown at this point.

Creatine-Transport Powders Boost Uptake

In 1996, a study at Queens Medical Centre in Nottingham, England, compared creatine retention in twenty-two healthy men. Researchers divided the men into four groups. Group A took 5 g of creatine, Groups B and C consumed 5 g of creatine with 93 g of simple sugar (creatine-carb mixture), and Group D took an inert substance technically called a placebo. All groups took their supplements four times per day. In addition, Group C rode stationary bikes for an hour each day, while the other groups did not exercise.

The researchers found that the creatine-carb mixture boosted total muscle-creatine levels 24 percent by day three, while creatine alone produced only a 14 percent increase. Furthermore, although exercise normally increases creatine retention, the added carbs were so effective that there was no difference between the creatine levels in Groups B and C.

This study led to the introduction of several creatine-transport powders. All of these supplements include simple sugars (usually dextrose but sometimes maltose or maltodextrin) in varying amounts along with other ingredients that have anabolic properties, such as the amino acids taurine and glutamine. They come in lemon-lime, orange, grape, and fruit-punch flavors.

Some products have nutrients that may further boost creatine uptake and retention. The antioxidant alpha-lipoic acid has been shown to increase insulin sensitivity in people with diabetes. Since insulin is involved in creatine uptake, alpha-lipoic acid may therefore help deliver creatine to the muscle cells.

Arginine increases blood flow to the penis, which is why it is included in "male health" products. Logically, it should increase blood flow to other muscles as well, permitting more nutrients (including creatine) to be transported. However, no studies have been published that specifically show enhanced creatine uptake from alpha-lipoic acid or arginine. On the other hand, a recent study did show increased uptake with D-pinitol, a nutrient found in pine wood and legumes.

Another study compared pure carbs with a 50/50 protein-carb blend and found that creatine uptake was the same in both cases. As a result, you can add protein powder to your creatine-transport drink without any reduction in benefit. Given the need for amino acids before and after your workout, this is a very good idea.

Effervescent Creatine: The Fizz That Builds Muscle

Recently, numerous effervescent creatine powders have been introduced. When combined with water, these powders provide an effective dose of creatine in a bubbly, flavorful beverage. A well-designed effervescent creatine increases the solubility of creatine, so less is left in the glass and more can reach the bloodstream and muscle cells.

Although some brands use creatine monohydrate, most effervescent creatine is made with creatine citrate. Sometimes, citric and/or ascorbic acid are also added to the mix. The addition of these acidic ingredients lowers the pH of the drink, which has been shown to increase the amount of creatine that dissolves in water.

Sodium carbonate and/or bicarbonate combines with the citric and/or ascorbic acid to produce the effervescence, while various sweeteners, such as dextrose, fructose, stevia, aspartame, and acesulfame-K, reduce the extreme tartness of the creatine citrate. Natural sweeteners, particularly dextrose, help to increase the uptake of creatine, although, of course, the artificial sweeteners do not. Effervescent creatine is available in four flavors: orange, grape, fruit punch, and berry.

It's funny how things change as our knowledge expands. When creatine was first introduced, the locker-room talk was that you shouldn't mix it with orange juice because it would neutralize the effect. Now we know that the opposite is true: Not only does the acid in orange juice not neutralize it, it can actually enhance its solubility.

Effervescent creatine is a lot more enjoyable than downing creatine with water. This taste advantage is a big reason why these powders are so popular. However, there is no published evidence that effervescent creatine citrate increases the amount of creatine that makes it to the bloodstream compared with an equivalent amount of creatine monohydrate. Hopefully, future research will clarify this question.

Liquid Creatine: Revolutionary Discovery or Hoax?

Liquid creatine is the most controversial form of creatine on the market. While creatine monohydrate and creatine citrate are very stable compounds in dry form, nearly all scientists believe that they begin to degrade when dissolved in water. They wind up largely as creatinine, a harmless substance that is also the natural byproduct of creatine metabolism. Unfortunately, creatinine has zero anabolic properties.

This process begins after several hours, so there

is no reason to be concerned when you mix creatine or an effervescent formulation with water and drink it immediately. However, it does become an issue when the creatine is packaged in liquid form.

Liquid-creatine products contain ample amounts of creatine when they leave the factory. However, the products sit at a distributor for some time before being shipped to stores. They then spend time on store shelves before eventually being purchased. How much active ingredient is still there for the consumer is a topic of much debate.

"We've tried all sorts of ways to stabilize creatine in solution," says Joan Dean, a representative for SKW, the leading German manufacturer of creatine monohydrate. "We have one of the best laboratories in the world, and it can't be done."

Yet, billion-dollar, multinational corporations do not have a monopoly on wisdom and invention. Perhaps there is a Thomas Edison of creatine out there who has unlocked the mystery of stabilizing creatine in liquid. This revolutionary discovery would certainly make it more convenient to use creatine by eliminating the need to mix it with water or other liquid before taking it.

However, there is no peer-reviewed research on the content of liquid creatine purchased by athletes, and independent lab results put the creatine content at around 10 percent of the amount on the label. Also, no study has been performed comparing the anabolic potential of liquid creatine with the powdered forms.

Given the millions of dollars that are spent advertising liquid creatine each year, one would think that Mr. Edison would want to spend the $20,000 needed to do a clinical trial verifying its benefits. Alas, this has not occurred. You can draw your own conclusions.

Dosage Recommendations

Traditionally, athletes took 20–30 g per day for five

to seven days (know as a loading phase), followed by 4–7 g daily (maintenance phase). This was based on early research that showed it was an effective way to maximize muscle-creatine concentrations. And it is highly effective—as long as you can handle the possible side effects.

While the body can easily assimilate small amounts of creatine, if you take too much, you can overload your intestines and suffer the consequences, including gas and diarrhea. If you can't wait a month to get the full effects of creatine, then do a loading phase but stay close to a bathroom until you see how your body responds. (Some people have no problem at all with loading.)

However, if you don't mind waiting a month or don't want to take a chance with side effects, simply start with the old-style maintenance phase. Studies have shown that this dosage is perfectly capable of giving you all that creatine has to offer in thirty days without the downside.

The 4–7 g recommendation is valid for creatine monohydrate and citrate, regardless of the delivery system. Athletes who train intensely should aim for 7 g per day, while weekend warriors need only 4 g. Also, because creatine stores are related to muscle mass, larger athletes need more creatine to make the greatest gains.

Some athletes believe that doing on and off cycles with creatine is a must, while others say they experience no benefit. If you decide to give your body a "break," remember that it takes a full four weeks after you stop supplementing for creatine levels to return to normal. Cycling one day on/one day off or even one week on/one week off is therefore pointless.

Also, since there is a maximum creatine concentration in muscle tissue, once you get there, you can't exceed this physiological limit with cycling or anything else. Cycling will allow you to feel the great pump you felt when you first started taking creatine, but only because you lost its benefits during the time off. It's your choice.

Creatine is a relatively inexpensive supplement with an excellent cost-benefit ratio. Its effectiveness has been verified beyond a shadow of a doubt, as has its safety. (Rumors about cramping and dehydration have proved unfounded.) If you haven't given creatine a try, you definitely should.

CHAPTER 3

GLUTAMINE AND OTHER SECRETAGOGUES

Growth hormone (GH) is one of the most important hormones for the athlete. While testosterone gets most of the attention, GH does much of the work in increasing your strength and muscle mass. GH has a major role in muscle growth and retention due to its ability to promote cell division and proliferation throughout the body. It enhances protein synthesis and nitrogen retention, and stimulates the liver to produce various growth factors. GH also promotes the growth of the bones and connective tissues, as well as enhancing the rate of healing. It even reduces body-fat levels by raising your metabolic rate and increasing the use of fats as an energy source.

Because of these many roles, you can't train and perform at your peak unless you have an ample supply of GH. Teenagers and young adults tend to have enough, which is part of the reason they grow so quickly. Older individuals have less and less each year. While bioengineered GH is available, it requires a prescription, which can be obtained only if you are extremely deficient in this hormone. This has led supplement manufacturers to develop a number of GH boosters, known as *secretagogues*, to help you increase your supply of this essential hormone.

Secretagogue
An amino acid or other substance that stimulates a gland of your body to secrete a particular hormone.

This chapter discusses the most common secretagogues for growth hormone. Some, like glutamine and arginine, are amino acids, while others are brain chemicals or precursors to these chemicals. All help your pituitary gland to release more GH.

Glutamine: An Important Amino Acid

Scientists have known about glutamine for decades, but it was written off as "just" an amino acid for many years. Since the body can produce glutamine under normal conditions from other amino acids, glutamine has been called a nonessential amino acid—even though it has many essential roles in the body. However, when you are sick or under a great deal of stress, recent research has shown that these supplies of glutamine can be insufficient to meet all your body's needs.

Due to their increased activity levels and metabolic requirements, athletes can develop relative deficiencies of glutamine that can hold back their training progress. In these situations, glutamine supplementation can remove a limiting factor and help the athlete to achieve his or her optimal performance.

Glutamine is the most abundant amino acid in the human body. The majority of this glutamine is stored within the skeletal muscles, although significant amounts are also found in the blood, lungs, liver, and brain. The cells of the immune system use glutamine for fuel (most of the body's cells use glucose). In addition, glutamine provides fuel for the mucosal cells of the intestinal wall, which helps to promote the maximum assimilation of vital nutrients for athletic activity.

Because it has a nitrogen atom to spare, glutamine is able to transport nitrogen around the body. This "shuttle" activity helps it to neutralize the lactic acid that builds up during exercise. The greater the availability of glutamine, the quicker this lactic acid can be neutralized. This can allow exercise to resume sooner and may even permit higher strength levels during your workout. Glutamine also acts as a nitrogen precursor for several coenzymes and the phosphate molecules that muscles use for energy production.

This amino acid plays a role in the maintenance of protein balance in muscle by increasing protein synthesis and reducing protein breakdown. The more glutamine in the muscle cells, the higher the rate of protein synthesis. This is because glutamine increases the amount of fluid inside the muscle cell, which is a powerful anabolic signal for the building of new proteins. This volumization is similar to (but not as strong as) that produced by creatine.

A Proven Growth-Hormone Booster

A study at Louisiana State University found that oral glutamine supplementation had a dramatic impact on growth-hormone secretion. Nine healthy volunteers aged thirty-two to sixty-four consumed 2 g of glutamine over a twenty-minute period that started forty-five minutes after a light breakfast. During the next ninety minutes, blood samples were measured every half-hour for plasma GH and the level of bicarbonate, which is a salt that can reduce acid levels in the body.

The researchers found that GH levels rose 430 percent above baseline levels after ninety minutes. There was a dramatic rise in bicarbonate concentration as well, which could help neutralize the lactic acid produced during a workout.

To stimulate your GH secretion, you should consume 2 to 3 g of glutamine with a glass of water several times per day. Tomas Welbourne, the author of this study, notes that high blood-sugar levels prevent glutamine from promoting GH release, so be sure to take it at least one hour after a meal or one hour before your next one.

Also, Welbourne recommends that you don't exceed a 3-g dose, because greater amounts could be counterproductive for GH production. Larger dosages, however, have proved effective for immune enhancement.

Glutamine Enhances Immunity

Strenuous exercise taxes your immune system. There is a higher incidence of infections and cold symptoms after a bout of intense exercise. Researchers at the University of Oxford found that there is a decrease in the plasma level of glutamine in endurance athletes after a marathon. This reduction continues for one hour, then slowly returns to normal sixteen hours after the event.

During this period, there is also a drop in the number of lymphocytes (white blood cells), which are dependent on glutamine for optimal growth. The decline in lymphocyte count, along with other negative changes in the immune system, is considered by many researchers to be the cause of the increased frequency of illness among athletes.

Here again, glutamine can help. Researchers at Oxford and the Free University of Brussels found a correlation between oral glutamine consumption and the absence of illness in trained athletes. They measured the levels of infection in more than 200 runners and rowers. Middle-distance runners had the lowest infection rate, while the rowers and full- or ultra-marathon runners had the highest levels.

The researchers then gave a total of 5 g of glutamine to half of these athletes while the others drank a placebo. Half of the dosage was taken right after the exercise bout and the remainder was consumed two hours after exercise. The results were dramatic. Only 19 percent of the athletes using glutamine reported infections during the next seven days, while 51 percent of the athletes on the placebo came down with a cold or similar infection. Given how frustrated athletes get when they are forced to take time off, supplementation with glutamine is great health insurance.

Best Supplementation Regimen

Even though the body produces 50–120 g of glutamine on its own each day, supplementation has been shown to provide additional benefits. While part of your dose winds up being metabolized by the mucosal cells of the small intestine, it is still beneficial because the body uses this external source instead of getting the glutamine it needs from your muscles (the main storage area for this amino acid).

You can minimize this drain on your muscle stores by taking 5 g of glutamine right before your workout. This will help to reduce lactic-acid concentrations during exercise as well. You should also take 5 g after your workout to speed up your recovery. While these larger doses may not stimulate GH production, they will help to keep your body in a positive glutamine balance and minimize any negative impact from your training. This by itself may help the pituitary gland to release more GH on its own. To maximize glutamine's benefits, take an additional 2 to 3 g between meals to bump up your GH level.

Arginine Has Many Important Functions

Arginine is another amino acid that is considered nonessential because the body can normally produce enough of it. However, as with glutamine, dietary deprivation, trauma, severe stress, and other conditions can create arginine deficiencies.

This amino acid has a variety of vital functions. It is used for the synthesis of many proteins and is the only source for a chemical group used by the body to manufacture creatine. (Lysine and methionine provide the other chemical raw materials.) It promotes wound healing and is found in large amounts in semen.

Arginine is involved in the regulation of nitric oxide. Elevated levels of nitric oxide dilate the arteries and increase blood flow. This boosts the volume of nutrients delivered to the target tissues, which is why some supplement companies include arginine in their creatine-transport drinks or other products.

Arginine is also required for the detoxification of

ammonia, which is formed during the metabolism of amino acids, nucleic acids, and other substrates that contain nitrogen. Since the average body produces 3–4 g of ammonia each day, adequate arginine intake is clearly important.

How to Get a GH Release

Arginine is found in relatively high quantities in chicken, turkey, and nuts. However, supplementation is needed to get an increase in growth-hormone levels. Some researchers have reported positive effects from as little as 5–10 g of arginine per day, although most studies have used larger dosages (up to 30 g). The amino acid has normally been taken right before bedtime on an empty stomach so it can increase the amount of GH released during sleep, which is when the body secretes the greatest amount of this hormone. Why you need to take more arginine than glutamine to get results is not clear at this point.

A study at the Rome Medical Clinic in Italy found that a combination of arginine and lysine dramatically increased GH levels at a much smaller dose. The test subjects took 1,200 mg of arginine pyro - glutamate and 1,200 mg of lysine hydrochloride. Within ninety minutes of taking this supplement, GH levels rose 700 percent above baseline levels. Eight hours later, GH levels were still elevated by as much as 300 percent. These dosage levels are more in line with those required for GH release with glutamine. Apparently, the combination with lysine and/or the form of arginine used made the difference.

Arginine is usually a very safe amino acid. However, if you have herpes simplex or suffer from schizophrenia, you should avoid using arginine, since it could worsen your condition. Choose a different secretagogue instead.

Other Effective Secretagogues

Many researchers believe that you can boost GH

levels by increasing the concentrations of the neurotransmitters acetylcholine and dopamine.

Like most hormones, the levels of these neurotransmitters decrease as you get older. A precursor to acetylcholine, alpha-glycerylphosphorylcholine, has been shown to stimulate GH secretion by reducing the amount of somatostatin (GH-inhibiting hormone) that is released.

Neurotransmitters
Brain chemicals that have a number of important roles in your brain. They regulate everything from emotions and muscle movement to tissue growth and repair.

L-dopa, an amino acid that the brain uses to make dopamine, is an effective secretagogue. Made popular by Durk Pearson and Sandy Shaw in their best-seller *Life Extension,* L-dopa was reported to increase GH output at a dose of 500 mg per day. L-dopa is produced naturally by the body through the oxidation of the amino acid tyrosine. Available as a prescription drug, L-dopa is also found in the herb *Mucuna pruriens* and in fava beans. *Bacopa monniera* is sometimes added to these neurotransmitter-based formulas because the bacosides it contains help to repair damaged neurons.

A study at Walsh University gave a single dose of a botanical supplement containing 666 mg of *Mucuna pruriens*, 100 mg of alpha glycerylphosphorylcholine, and 50 mg of *Bacopa monniera* to five young men thirty minutes before performing six sets of squats. The researchers found that total GH levels were 19.8 percent higher during the sixty-minute recovery period, while peak GH levels increased nearly 90 percent.

Another way to stimulate your GH release is to use homeopathic products. Homeopathy is a branch of medicine that uses highly diluted concentrations of certain substances to trigger a response by the body. In this case, it is believed that a small amount of GH will cause the pituitary gland to secrete more GH.

Homeopathy has many followers, but the FDA is not one of them. It considers such diluted doses to be useless (although harmless), and therefore permits real growth hormone to be sold over the counter as long as the amount of GH in the pill is small enough. There is little research on these products, so you'll need to experiment and see what results you get for yourself.

With the increasing recognition of growth hormone's many contributions to sports performance, more and more athletes are using GH secretagogues. They can be valuable additions to your supplement regimen, but don't go overboard with them. The pituitary gland and the brain are complex organs with many feedback loops, so stick with the manufacturers' recommendations. That way you can get all of the benefits of this vital hormone.

CHAPTER 4

VITAMINS AND MINERALS

Athletes need to be sure that they consume sufficient vitamins and minerals. These micronutrients play vital roles in muscle development, energy production, and many other essential functions. While they are often taken for granted, vitamins and minerals enable you to perform at your peak.

Your micronutrient requirements go up as the intensity of your training increases, so you want to be sure you get enough. At the same time, taking more than you need is expensive and does not provide any additional sports benefit.

This chapter is limited to the role of vitamins and minerals in enhancing your performance as an athlete. While these nutrients can provide many additional health benefits, these topics are outside the scope of this book. For a detailed look at the micro - nutrients, check out *User's Guide to Vitamins and Minerals* by Jack Challem & Liz Brown (Basic Health Publications, 2002).

Vitamins Are Needed for Chemical Reactions

There are currently thirteen vitamins that are recognized as essential for humans: vitamin A (retinol), B_1 (thiamin), B_2 (riboflavin), B_3 (niacin), B_6 (pyridoxine), B_{12} (cobalamin), pantothenic acid, folic acid, biotin, C, D, E, and K. Even though your body's requirements for these nutrients are small compared with the macronutrients (protein, carbs, and fat), a deficiency of any one of them can lead to illness and disease.

Vitamins

Nutrients that are required for many different chemical reactions within the body. They help regulate the chain of metabolic reactions that controls tissue synthe - sis, the release of energy in food, and other functions.

Without the right vitamins, essential chemical reactions cannot take place at the proper rates, impacting your body's metabolic processes. Some vitamins also act as antioxidants, helping to pro- tect you from potentially cancer-causing compounds called free radicals.

There are two types of vitamins: fat-soluble and water-soluble. The fat-soluble vitamins (A, D, E, and K) can be dissolved only in fat. A small amount of fat must therefore be included in the diet so that these vitamins can be assimilated and used by the body. Fat-soluble vita- mins that are not immediately needed are stored in the fat tissues for later use, so deficiencies of fat-soluble vitamins are relatively rare.

In fact, because these vitamins remain in the sys- tem for so long, athletes who take extremely high amounts of fat-soluble vitamins can actually devel- op toxic levels in their bodies. For this reason, care should be taken when consuming fat-soluble vita- min supplements.

The water-soluble vitamins (B-complex vitamins and vitamin C) act as coenzymes. They combine with small protein molecules to form active enzymes. These vitamins dissolve in water but not in fat. As a result, they cannot be stored to any great degree by the body. Water-soluble vitamin supplies that are not immediately needed are likely to be excreted in the urine. It is therefore necessary to eat foods and supplements that contain these vitamins on a regular basis to prevent deficiencies.

Minerals Build a Strong Body

Minerals are also required for sports performance. There are twenty-two minerals that are currently rec- ognized as essential: calcium, phosphorus, sulfur, potassium, chlorine, sodium, magnesium, iron, fluorine, zinc, copper, selenium, iodine, chromium, cobalt, silicon, vanadium, tin, nickel, manganese, molybdenum, and lead.

While vitamins are able to facilitate chemical reactions in the body without actually becoming part of them, minerals usually become incorporated within the body's physical and chemical structures. Minerals are found in the body's enzymes and hormones, too. They regulate the acid-base balance of the body, help control cellular metabolism, and stimulate various reactions that allow energy to be released from the foods we eat.

Minerals

Metals, some of which play an essential role in formation of the teeth and bones. Minerals are also involved in functions as diverse as maintaining a normal heartbeat, allowing the muscles to contract and relax, and permitting the nerves to transmit impulses.

Minerals have been divided into two groups, known as major minerals and trace minerals, depending on the quantity of the mineral you need. Individual minerals also vary in the degree to which the body absorbs them. This variation, called bioavailability, can range from as low as 5 percent for manganese to 30 to 40 percent for calcium and magnesium. The bioavailability of a mineral is taken into consideration when the daily value for that mineral is established.

It should be noted that the levels of toxicity for minerals are much lower than they are for vitamins. This is because minerals are metals, so they should be treated with a great deal of respect. Taking too many minerals can definitely harm your health without giving you any performance benefit in return.

Daily Requirements for Athletes

Athletes tend to eat relatively large quantities of good food. This dietary intake should provide a substantial portion of your total vitamin and mineral requirements. In some cases, it may supply all of an athlete's needs for a particular micronutrient. Also, bear in mind that vitamins have the ability to be used over and over in metabolic reactions, so there is not a direct correlation between activity levels and vitamin needs. Still, many athletes require additional micronutrients to perform at their best. This can be achieved by taking a multivitamin/multimineral supplement that contains the daily value for each micronutrient once or twice a day depending on how nutritious your meals are.

There are four micronutrients that are particularly important for muscle growth and sports performance: vitamin C, vitamin E, calcium, and magnesium. Several studies have shown sports benefits from these nutrients at levels significantly greater than the daily value, so you should take extra amounts of them in addition to your multivitamin/multimineral supplement.

Vitamins C and E Fight Free Radicals

Vitamin C is well known for its ability to help strengthen the immune system. This antioxidant vitamin can also help neutralize potentially damaging free radicals, which have been connected with a number of diseases. Researchers at the University of Cape Town, South Africa, gave 600 mg of the vitamin to the participants of a ninety-kilometer race. They found that supplementation significantly reduced the incidence of common cold symptoms during this acute physical stress.

Other placebo-controlled studies have shown that 1–2 g of vitamin C per day can decrease the severity of common cold symptoms. Therefore, in order to keep your immune system in peak condition, you should consume 1–2 g of vitamin C each day. Citrus fruits, tomatoes, green peppers, and green leafy vegetables contain good amounts of this vitamin. If you do not get enough from your diet, inexpensive tablets are available.

Vitamin E is another antioxidant vitamin. It is fat-soluble and is found primarily in cell membranes. Vitamin E helps to prevent free-radical damage in the muscles and bloodstream. It protects the red blood cells as well, and plays an essential role in cellular respiration in cardiac and skeletal muscle, which increases endurance and stamina.

Vitamin E also reduces the membrane disruption that occurs in exercised muscles due to increased free-radical production. A placebo-controlled study at Pennsylvania State University gave 1,200 IU of vitamin E to six weight-trained males for two weeks. The men were then asked to perform a vigorous whole-body workout after a two-day rest period. Vitamin E supplementation significantly reduced the muscle damage created by this workout program.

You should consume 600–1,200 IU of vitamin E per day. Good food sources include grains, green leafy vegetables and seeds. Many oils contain vitamin E as well, but you may prefer to take a supplement to keep your calorie count down.

Calcium Builds Strong Bones and Muscles

Calcium is the most abundant mineral in the human body. It assists in regulating the heartbeat and helps to build and maintain the bones and teeth. Calcium reduces lactic-acid concentrations in the blood during and after exercise. It is also essential for muscle contraction.

When a muscle fiber is stimulated to contract, calcium binds to one of the protein-based filaments deep inside the muscle cell, and, in effect, turns it on. When the nerve impulse to the muscle fiber is removed, the calcium ions move back to their storage location, which stops the contraction of the muscle.

In order to ensure an adequate calcium supply, you should consume 7 mg of calcium per pound of

body weight (16 mg/kg). Good food sources of calcium include nonfat milk and yogurt, mozzarella
cheese, broccoli, and green leafy vegetables. If you
don't get enough from your diet, you should buy
calcium carbonate or calcium citrate tablets to make
up the difference. These forms of calcium are more
bioavailable than the less expensive bone-meal or
oyster-shell products.

Magnesium Activates Many Enzymes

Magnesium helps to control carbohydrate synthesis and is an essential activator of many enzyme
systems. It counteracts the stimulatory effect of
calcium in the muscle fibers and helps to prevent
muscle cramps. A study at the University of North
Dakota found that it enhances oxygen delivery to
working muscles in trained subjects. Magnesium
supplementation has also been shown to reduce
the level of hormones that can produce a loss of
muscle tissue.

Despite its importance, the body contains less
than an ounce (20 g) of magnesium, 27 percent of
which is found in muscle. You should consume
3.5 mg of magnesium per pound of body weight
(8 mg/kg). There are not many good food sources
of magnesium except for cod, snapper, and some
other seafood. Whole grains and vegetables contain small amounts. Fortunately, magnesium tablets
are inexpensive.

By providing your body with a balanced spec-
trum of micronutrients, you ensure that no vitamin
or mineral becomes a limiting factor in your muscle
growth. Given the moderate expense involved, you
should make sure that you get enough vitamins and
minerals every day.

CHAPTER 5

ECDYSTERONE

During the Cold War, there were plenty of rumors about the "secret" training techniques of athletes in the former Soviet Union. Depending on who was doing the telling, they were all jacked up on anabolic steroids, subjected to bizarre training programs, underwent psychological brainwashing, or all of the above. Lost in the hysteria was the use by Soviet athletes of benign, but effective, natural substances like ecdysterone and related ecdysteroids.

An Adaptogen That Works

The Russians who dominated the USSR have been big believers in the power of herbs for a long time. While scoffed at by American researchers who think that only refined pharmaceuticals hold any value, the Russians have experimented with herbs for dec-ades. Their main focus has been on adaptogenic herbs, which are plants that have the ability to restore optimal function in athletes who are depleted because of their training.

Adaptogen
An herb that has a variable effect depending on your physical condition. The further you are from an optimal state, the more benefit you receive.

The concept of adaptogens can be difficult for Americans to understand, but it is well recognized in Asia and even in Europe, where herbs play a much greater role in medicine than in this country. If you are in prime condition already, you may not see much of a change from using adaptogenic herbs. However, if you are overtrained or depleted in some way, as athletes often are, you may see a significant change for the better.

Once the Iron Curtain fell, Westerners learned about the effectiveness of *Rhaponticum carthamoides*, also known as *Leuzea carthamoides*. This herb is a perennial that grows in Central Asia. Long recognized as a rejuvenator and metabolic stimulant in local folklore, scientists discovered that it contains a high concentration of ecdysteroids, especially 20-hydroxyecdysone (20-E).

Ecdysteroids Are Widespread

There are about 200 members in the ecdysteroid family, all of which are chemically related to 20-E. These ecdysteroids are widespread in plants and even in insects. In fact, ecdysteroids are the steroid hormones of invertebrates, functioning much as testosterone does in man. Ecdysteroids regulate many biochemical and physiological processes in insects, including maturation and reproduction.

The role of ecdysteroids in plants is still unclear, although they are thought to help protect the plant from insect damage. Concentrations are highest in the parts of the plant that are most important to its survival. In many species, 20-E is the most common ecdysteroid, and it is considered to be the most biologically active of these compounds.

A review of thousands of plant species has revealed that *Rhaponticum carthamoides* has the highest proportion of 20-E of any plant studied. However, *Pfaffia paniculata*, an herb found in the Brazilian rain forest, also contains 20-E in moderate amounts. This has led to a debate about whether the extracts of these plants provide the same benefits.

While the absence of research on *Pfaffia paniculata* makes it difficult to make a categorical statement, bear in mind that the other ecdysteroids in an herbal extract likely play a role in its effectiveness. Since nearly all of the available research is on

Rhaponticum carthamoides, it is your best bet at this time as a source of 20-E.

Among vegetables, spinach has the highest concentration of 20-E. Could this be the real reason that Popeye has such big arms?

Numerous Anabolic Properties

Because of their many plant sources, ecdysteroids are commonly found in humans in low concentrations. They pass through the acidic conditions of the stomach without apparent changes to their structure and are easily assimilated. Maximum levels in the blood occur thirty minutes to two hours after they are consumed, depending on whether food is eaten along with the ecdysteroids.

They are eliminated relatively quickly from the blood. Ecdysone, a fairly common ecdysteroid, has a half-life of four hours, while 20-E has a half-life of nine hours.

A Half-Life
A measure of how long it takes for half of a substance to be degraded and eliminated by the body.

This suggests that you should take ecdysteroids several times per day to maintain high blood levels. Studies in mice indicate that the bioavailability is around 50 percent—fairly high for an herb.

Ecdysteroids have a number of anabolic properties. Several studies have shown a rise in protein synthesis with ecdysterone administration. A Japanese study found a 51 percent increase in protein levels when mice were given orally 5 mg of ecdy - steroids per kilogram of body weight. The increase in protein levels peaked two to four hours after ecdysterone administration. These results were confirmed by two Russian studies.

In all cases, the changes were largely due to an increase in ribosomal activity. Ribosomes are cellular proteins that hook amino acids together to form new proteins. Also detected was a greater amount of messenger ribonucleic acid, which the body uses as a template for protein synthesis.

Remember that your body can create new muscle proteins only if sufficient raw material is available. Therefore, be sure to eat plenty of dietary protein each day (at least 1 g per pound of body weight). This will provide an adequate supply of amino acids, which your ribosomes can then incorporate into new muscle proteins. And, of course, give it your all in the gym.

More Advantages for Athletes

Training is hard work, and if you do it right, it will drain you of energy. Increases in work capacity are therefore very helpful. The longer you can work out, the more likely you are to accomplish your sports goals.

Several Russian studies have found enhanced work capacity with ecdysteroids. A study with mice found that a *Rhaponticum carthamoides* extract increased swimming time by 22 percent, while the length of time the mice could run before exhaustion rose by 32 percent. A twenty-day study of forty-four athletes found a similar increase in working capacity, which was measured on a bicycle ergometer (a tool used to measure work performance). Unfortunately, information regarding the dosages used in these studies is not available.

Most athletes are interested in gaining muscular size and strength, and several studies suggest that ecdysterone can help. A study performed at the Czech Academy of Sciences found that 20-E was effective in increasing the growth rate of Japanese quail. These animals, which grow quickly anyway, packed on 7 percent more body mass than the control group in only four weeks when given 20 mg of 20-E per kilogram of body weight. This occurred despite the fact that the 20-E group ate less, indicating that this ecdysterone may increase the efficiency of food assimilation.

These studies show that ecdysteroids can be effective anabolic agents. Even better, toxicological studies show that ecdysteroids are very safe. Because they do not operate through hormonal pathways, ecdysteroids cannot cause the negative effects produced by anabolic steroids. This makes them a much better choice for long-term use.

Other Health-Related Benefits

Ecdysteroids have other benefits as well. A study published in *Eksperimentalnaia i Klinicheskaia Farmakologiia* found that ecdysterone enhanced the sex function and behavioral characteristics of rats, especially in the first few days. The scientists, who gave the rats 5 mg of ecdysterone per kilogram of body weight each day for ten days, also found that it increased copulative function and improved the quality of their sperm.

Other experiments have shown that ecdysteroids have antioxidant properties, reducing the oxidation of LDL cholesterol (the so-called "bad" cholesterol) in both test-tube and animal studies. Ecdysteroids have also stimulated immune function in mice at a dosage of 5–20 mg/kg (milligrams per kilogram). In addition, a study on sixty Soviet cadets and forty-seven sailors found increased appetite and an improved mental state from an ecdysteroid extract. These studies support the traditional use of *Rhaponticum carthamoides* as a rejuvenator.

With such an extensive array of benefits, it is no wonder that ecdysterone and related ecdysteroids have become part of the supplement regimen of many athletes. They promote protein synthesis, boost work capacity, and increase muscle mass. As with all herbs, be sure to consider the dosages given in the studies and take the same amounts. And for maximum effect, choose an extract with a high concentration of 20-E. When used appropriately, ecdysteroids can be a valuable addition to your training program.

CHAPTER 6

GINSENG AND ASTRAGALUS

Ginseng is one of the most popular herbs in the world, while astragalus is relatively unknown in Western countries. Both of these herbs have important benefits for the athlete, ranging from increased endurance and strength to enhanced immune function. Like *Rhaponticum carthamoides,* ginseng and astragalus work through nonhormonal pathways, so they can be used for extended periods. But it takes a while for you to see noticeable effects.

Ginseng has been the subject of a wide variety of research experiments in Western countries, both in animals and in humans. The results of these studies are all over the board for reasons that are discussed in this chapter. Nearly all of the experiments with astragalus have been done in China, where the herb is even more popular than ginseng. The bottom line from these studies is that ginseng and astragalus will help you perform better in your sport—pro - vided that you take enough of a standardized extract for a long enough time.

The Many Types of Ginseng

While ginseng is often considered a single plant, there are actually three to nine types of ginseng depending on who's counting. The three most popular ginsengs are *Panax ginseng* (Chinese or Korean ginseng), *Panax quinquefolius* (American ginseng), and *Eleutherococcus senticosus* (Siberian ginseng). Virtually all of the research in humans has been done with *Panax ginseng,* which is the most stimulating of the ginseng varieties.

The other plants that are similar to these ginsengs are *Panax pseudoginseng* (Tienqi ginseng), *Panax japonica* (Japanese ginseng), *Codonopsis pilosula* (False ginseng), *Pseudostellaria heterophylla* (Prince's ginseng), *Angelica sinensis* (dong quai), and *Glehnia littoralis* (glehnia root). As you can tell from the botanical names, several of these "ginsengs" aren't even in the same plant family as the Panax varieties.

Be sure to look at the label on your ginseng supplement to see which herb it contains. The non-Panax ginsengs are much weaker than the real thing, so you could be paying for a cheap imitation. If the supplement does not specify which ginseng it contains, choose a different product.

The King of Herbs

Panax ginseng has been revered in China as the King of Herbs for centuries. It is said to replenish the *qi*, or life force, of the body through a number of mechanisms. *Panax ginseng* works with the body to help restore balance. Chinese practitioners use it as a tonic to increase physical strength and energy and to promote the proper functioning of the body's organs. They also use it to treat fatigue.

Panax ginseng builds stamina and endurance by enhancing the body's ability to adapt to stress, and it was used extensively in former Soviet countries as a way to boost strength and athletic performance. (Siberian ginseng and *Rhaponticum carthamoides* were also used for these purposes.)

A number of animal studies have confirmed these benefits. A placebo-controlled study at the University of Alberta with rats not accustomed to exercise found a significant increase in VO_{2max} after four days of ginseng saponin injections.

VO_{2max}
A measure of aerobic fitness. It measures the maximum volume of oxygen (O_2) that your lungs can hold.

Ginseng treatment also significantly increased

the amount of free fatty acids in the blood and preserved glucose levels during exercise. These alterations are favorable for the athlete, as they allow you to burn more fat and keep you from "hitting the wall" due to low glucose levels. The end result in greater exercise endurance.

A study published in *Ethnopharmacology* gave 100 mg/kg of an aqueous ginseng extract to mice orally for seven days. *Panax ginseng* produced a significant increase in swimming time compared with the control group. There was also an increase in body weight and in the mass of the *levator ani muscle,* the muscle that forms the floor of the pelvic cavity. (This was the only muscle studied.) In addition, an experiment at Toyama Medical and Pharmaceutical University with aged rats found that 8 g/kg per day of extract given orally for twelve days increased their performance in learning their way through a maze.

Proven Effectiveness in Humans

These animal studies, and most of the others before them, showed that *Panax ginseng* was effective in enhancing performance in rodents. Logically, scientists would then turn to human studies using the same relative amounts of ginseng to determine the effects in humans. However, in most cases this did not occur.

The animal studies that give the herb orally used a minimum of 100 mg per kilogram of body weight. The average human weighs 80 kg (176 lb). This means that an equivalent dose for a human would be 8,000 mg (or 8 g, a bit less than a third of an ounce). Yet most of the human studies used 200 mg of standardized extract (usually 4 percent ginsenosides), or 2.5 mg/kg. Surprise, surprise, these studies showed that ginseng didn't work! Whether these researchers were excessively conservative, out to show that the herbs didn't work, or simply clueless is unknown.

When appropriate levels of *Panax ginseng* are given for long enough periods, they consistently show the effectiveness of this herb. A six-week placebo-controlled study published in *International al Clinical Nutrition Review* gave 1,000 mg of ginseng root powder per day to fifteen men and fifteen women. Compared with the placebo, *Panax ginseng* significantly improved VO_{2max}. The heart rate of the test subjects was six beats per minute lower for the six minutes after exercise, suggesting improved recovery from the workout. Even better, pectoral strength increased by 22 percent, while quadriceps strength rose 18 percent. There was, however, no significant increase in grip strength.

A Danish study gave 400 mg of standardized extract to 112 healthy volunteers for eight to nine weeks. The researchers noted faster reaction times among the participants. Also, an abstract presented at the XXIII FIMS World Congress of Sports Medicine Abstracts noted improved endurance, VO_{2max}, post-exercise recovery, and simple reaction time in a study of 214 individuals. Unfortunately, the length of this study and the dosage given to the volunteers were not reported.

The Other Ginsengs

There has not been as much research into the benefits of the other ginsengs. *Panax quinquefolius* (American ginseng) is used as a tonic and natural stress reducer. According to practitioners of traditional Chinese medicine, it also helps to build *qi*, or life force, although it is less stimulatory than *Panax ginseng*. American ginseng promotes strength by increasing immunity through several mechanisms.

Curiously, American ginseng is more popular in China than in this country. Most of the U.S. crop is exported to Asia, where *Panax quinquefolius* has a reputation as an aphrodisiac. American ginseng is sometimes combined with *Panax ginseng* to produce an herbal blend that can boost energy levels while still relieving stress.

Siberian ginseng (*Eleutherococcus senticosus*) is not even from the same plant family as the Panax varieties. However, it does have some of the same stimulating and tonic effects as the other ginsengs. Like *Rhaponticum carthamoides*, it is native to Russia and has been used for generations to boost the strength and stamina of that country's athletes.

A study at two Japanese universities gave 300 mg per day of Siberian ginseng extract to six males to determine its effect on work capacity. This single-blind, cross-over study found significant increases in total work and time to exhaustion compared with the placebo group following eight days of supplementation. The researchers concluded that the improvements were due to changes in the participants' metabolisms, noting that VO_{2max} also increased.

No study to date has compared the benefits of *Panax ginseng* with American or Siberian ginseng. Also, there is virtually no research on the other types of ginseng. For now, you should avoid them. Stick with the proven winners.

Tips for Using Ginseng

Numerous studies have confirmed that ginseng can be of major benefit to athletes. Anything that increases your strength and aerobic potential while enhancing recovery and mental alertness will translate into significant gains in sports performance. However, you need to bear in mind that ginseng is an herb, not a prescription drug. As a result, you need to take a relatively large amount to get the results you want (although less than the dose for creatine or glutamine).

Always use a standardized root extract. Avoid products that are simply root powder and those that say only ginseng. If root is not specified, the manufacturer has probably substituted the less expensive (and less beneficial) leaves and branches of the plant. The root is where the highest concentrations of the active ingredients are found, so don't go simply by the milligrams per capsule. Buy the real thing.

The most beneficial chemicals in the plants are glycosylated steroidal saponins, usually referred to as ginsenosides. Thirteen different ginsenosides have been isolated so far, and each has specific properties. The most prevalent in *Panax ginseng* and *Panax quinquefolius* are R_b, R_c, and R_g, although their concentrations within these two herbs vary.

Because these ginsenosides interact with one another, herbal specialists recommend that a whole-root extract be used instead of a brand that only has a particular ginsenoside. Besides, at this point, we don't know enough about the properties of each one to be that precise. This remains a topic for future research.

How to Maximize Ginseng's Benefits

All extracts are standardized for total ginsenosides, so go for the strongest one you can get. The products currently on the market have a wide range of ginsenoside content. The most well-known product has 4 percent ginsenosides, although you can buy products with up to 10 percent ginsenosides. If the label does not mention the ginsenoside content, pick another brand. The manufacturer is not keeping you in the dark to save ink on the label, if you catch my drift.

Ideally, the extract will also include standardization for polysaccharides. This is because there are beneficial components in ginseng other than ginsenosides. Aim for a product that has 10 percent polysaccharides.

While the precise dosage depends on the percentage of ginsenosides and polysaccharides, you should consume a minimum of 500 mg of extract per day. Begin at this level and increase it to 750 mg and then 1,000 mg per day as needed. It is best to give your body time to adjust to this herbal extract. Also, take it for a minimum of three months before deciding whether you want to continue it for the long term. It takes time to achieve ginseng's benefits.

Astragalus: The Immune Booster

While largely unknown in Western countries, *Astragalus membranaceus* has been used for thousands of years in traditional Chinese medicine as part of the Fu Zheng therapy to enhance natural defense mechanisms.

Chinese herbalists have utilized astragalus to treat every type of fatigue and exhaustion. The herb is said to stabilize the exterior of the body and increase its resistance to disease by increasing the circulation of *wei qi,* or protective life force, on the body's surface. This enhances immune function and boosts the body's ability to adapt to stress.

What difference does this make for the athlete? Exercise is inherently stressful. The body is forced to perform intensely, which can reduce your resistance. Many an athlete has caught a cold or the flu because he or she trained so much that his or her body was susceptible to any bug that passed by. By fortifying your immune system, you can help to prevent these frustrating and strength-depleting episodes with illness.

Researchers have undertaken numerous experiments with astragalus to confirm its benefits using the tools of modern science. It has been shown to have a very strong antioxidant effect. The herb also stimulates the production of white blood cells, stem cells, macrophages, and lymphocytes, helping the immune system to hold off invading organisms and accelerating healing. Astragalus also helps to protect the liver from toxins, and it has even been shown to increase sperm motility.

A study in the *Japanese Journal of Hygiene* gave mice 200 mg/kg of astragalus per day. They were then forced to run at a rapid rate for sixty minutes five times per day for twelve weeks. The scientists found that astragalus intensified the functioning of their host defense systems, allowing them to tolerate the exercise regimen better.

Astragalus has many active components. Most are plant chemicals called astragalosides, seven of which have been isolated. Astragalus is also a natural source of methoxyisoflavone, which is discussed in Chapter 8. Each of these nutrients has a specific role, so you want to get a whole extract of the root. Various polysaccharides in astragalus have immune-stimulating properties as well.

As with ginseng, the astragalus products on the market have a wide variety of strengths. Only buy astragalus extracts, preferably water-based ones. Avoid products that just contain root powder. Aim for a flavonoid content of at least 1 percent and a polysaccharide content of 20 percent or more. This will ensure that you get an effective level of the active ingredients.

Synergy between Ginseng and Astragalus

Astragalus is frequently combined with ginseng in traditional Chinese medicine because of its synergistic actions with that herb. While ginseng stimulates the body's "aggressive" energy levels, astragalus strengthens the body's "defensive" energies, promoting a balance that gives you vitality without the jitters produced by most stimulants.

A recent study at Wichita State University examined the impact of a patented supplement that combines creatine with two forms of ginseng and astragalus (U.S. patent). Forty-four volunteers were divided into three groups. One group received a placebo, another took 3 g of creatine per day, and a third took 3 g of creatine plus 1,500 mg of an herbal extract that was 50 percent astragalus, 30 percent *Panax ginseng,* and 20 percent *Panax quinquefolius.*

The test subjects trained with weights for forty minutes three times per week for twelve weeks.

"The creatine/herbal blend produced statistically significant strength increases compared to placebo on all six exercises measured," noted lead researcher Dr. Michael Rogers. On the bench press, the subjects using this blend had strength increases that were three times greater than did those who took creatine alone. Vigor, as measured by the standardized Profile of Mood States, rose 18.9 percent. There were also dramatic increases in immune function.

These findings confirm that ginseng and astragalus are powerful herbs, especially when taken together. For maximum benefit, use a product that contains a single extract made from these herbs in the 50/30/20 ratio. This proven formulation will promote the greatest gains in your strength and sports performance.

CHAPTER 7

PHOSPHATIDYLSERINE

Physical exercise produces hormonal changes both during and after your workout. These hormones have a variety of impacts on the muscles and other tissues. Some of them are positive, helping the body to recuperate from the stresses of training. Others are negative, potentially keeping your body from recovering as quickly as you would like.

One of the hormones that can be negative is cortisol. Researchers have now found that phosphatidylserine (PS) can reduce cortisol levels, possibly promoting quicker recovery and growth.

Athletes try to reduce cortisol secretion because it suppresses the rate of protein formation and stimulates protein breakdown in tissues other than the liver. However, cortisol has other vital functions. It supports the action of hormones such as growth hormone and glucagon (which counteracts insulin and restores blood-sugar concentrations to normal levels). Cortisol also accelerates the release of stored fat and its use for energy, and even acts as an anti-inflammatory agent.

Cortisol
Cortisol is a hormone produced by the adrenal gland. It stimulates protein breakdown and can lead to a negative nitrogen balance when present in high concentrations over prolonged periods.

This means that the body often produces cortisol for a reason. As Thomas Fahey, Ph.D., professor of physical education at California State University, Chico, notes, "Suppressing cortisol levels a little bit is good because of its role in curbing protein synthesis. But you would never want to shut off its production entirely. It's there for a purpose!"

Benefits of This Essential Nutrient

Phosphatidylserine is an essential nutrient in our cells. It is one of a number of fat-based molecules that help to hold the cell membrane together. PS is particularly plentiful in nerve cells. Studies have shown that PS helps these cells to communicate with other cells by promoting the accumulation, storage, and release of neurotransmitters such as dopamine. This allows it to improve memory. PS also helps to transport nutrients into the cell and assists in the removal of waste products.

Scientists first looked at PS's ability to reduce cortisol levels with oral supplementation. A study at the University of Naples, Italy, gave 400 mg and 800 mg of PS to eight healthy males who performed an exercise protocol on a bicycle ergometer. The researchers found that 400 mg pf PS reduced cortisol levels in the blood by 16 percent, while 800 mg lowered cortisol concentrations by 25 percent.

Fahey and his associates conducted the second study. In this double-blind, cross-over study, ten trained weightlifters were given 800 mg of PS per day and then put through a vigorous whole-body workout four times per week that was intentionally designed to overtrain them. Each athlete received PS for two weeks, then repeated the workout program for another two weeks with the placebo after a three-week period in which no supplement was taken. Blood samples were taken fifteen minutes after their last workout on these two regimens and twenty-three hours after those workouts to see what the effects of overtraining were on their cortisol levels.

The study found that PS reduced postexercise cortisol levels by 20 percent. Exit interviews showed that the persons on PS "felt better" and had less muscle soreness. However, no differences in cortisol levels were found twenty-three hours after exercise. Apparently, the body is able to return cortisol levels to normal during this timeframe without supplemental PS.

Many Unknowns at This Point

These studies clearly show that PS can reduce cortisol levels when administered orally. However, we still don't know if cortisol production is a limiting factor in recuperation and muscle growth. "Science moves forward in small steps," notes Fahey. "First, we establish the correlation between cortisol and exercise, and then we investigate the implications of these findings."

So while researchers feel confident that PS reduces cortisol levels, they still don't know whether supplementation with PS will permit faster recovery or improve sports performance.

PS is found in only trace amounts in most foods. While the body is able to produce PS on its own, it must go through reactions that require a substantial amount of energy. This makes supplementation a better option.

Recommended Dosage and Side Effects

Phosphatidylserine is usually sold in 500-mg capsules or tablets containing a combination of PS and other phospholipids. Usually, about half of the total amount is PS. The standard dosage is two to three capsules per day, which would provide a daily dosage of PS approximately equal to the dose found effective in the clinical studies.

When PS is taken orally, it is rapidly absorbed. However, the single dosage of pure PS should be kept to around 250 mg for a couple of reasons. One, it's expensive. Two, in rare instances, dosages greater than this have been reported to cause nausea. This effect is minimized when PS is consumed with food. Also, don't take it right before going to bed, as the neurotransmitters it helps to release may make it harder for you to fall asleep. There do not appear to be any other side effects when taken at the recommended dosages.

In the future, PS may be considered a major anticatabolic nutrient. Until additional studies are completed, however, you'll need to do your own experiment and see what benefits you receive.

CHAPTER 8

METHOXYISOFLAVONE AND IPRIFLAVONE

In the last few years, a large number of products have been introduced that contain methoxyisoflavone and ipriflavone. Judging from the sales of these products, athletes seem to find them very effective. Unfortunately, these nutrients are so new that there isn't a lot of research on them, so you'll need to try them for yourself and see what improvements you get.

There Are Many Methoxyisoflavones

Flavones are naturally occurring substances found in fruits and vegetables. They have been shown to have a variety of positive health benefits when included in the diet, such as a decreased risk of various cancers. This has led scientists to look for the mechanisms behind these improvements.

Two test-tube studies have shown that biochanin A (5,7-dihydroxy-4-methoxyisoflavone) inhibits the activity of the enzyme aromatase, which converts testosterone to estrogen. While not the strongest reducer of aromatase levels out there, it does have a statistically significant level of activity. Another test-tube study showed that biochanin A mildly inhibits the 5-alpha-reductase enzyme. This enzyme converts testosterone to dihydrotestosterone, the form of the hormone largely responsible for the prostate problems most men experience later in life.

While soy is a good source of biochanin A, a study at the Institute of Endocrinology in Prague, Czech Republic, found that beer also contains this isoflavone, along with another called formononetin

(7-hydroxy-4-methoxyisoflavone). It's good to know that there are some beneficial nutrients in beer, but don't drink more because of it. Beer isn't exactly the breakfast of champions!

As you can see, there is more than one methoxy-isoflavone. (I'll skip the rest of the list.) However, the one that supplement manufacturers include in their formulations is 5-methyl-7-methoxyisoflavone—not biochanin A. This is important because claims are sometimes made for products using research on similar, but not identical, isoflavones.

The 5-methyl-7 Patent

The 5-methyl-7 form of methoxyisoflavone was first developed in Hungary, and a Budapest company received U.S. patent 4,163,746 for its efforts in 1979. This patent gave the company exclusive control over the invention until the mid-nineties, which is why methoxy products only started appearing on the market a few years ago.

In their patent application, the inventors stated that 5-methyl-7 increased the retention of calcium and phosphorous to a significant degree. In fact, one of the early uses for this compound and a related isoflavone called ipriflavone was as a treatment for osteoporosis. The inventors also noted that 5-methyl-7 increased nitrogen retention, which would lead to greater protein synthesis and consequent muscle growth. Unfortunately, the extent to which it enhanced protein synthesis was not revealed.

The patent did include the results of two studies on chickens. After five weeks, 5-methyl-7 increased the total body weight of chickens by 8 percent, while the weight of uncastrated cocks rose by 8.7 percent. These increases were primarily meat (muscle) and not fat.

No human studies were performed for this patent, much less studies with athletes. The inventors suggested, however, that an appropriate dose for humans would be 100 mg two or three times per day.

Good News about Ipriflavone

So where did all the claims you hear for methoxy-isoflavone come from? From an earlier patent on ipriflavone (7-isopropoxyisoflavone) by the same inventors. Like 5-methyl-7, ipriflavone is a synthetic isoflavone that does not work through hormonal pathways. Animal studies suggest that it has several benefits for athletes.

The inventors gave 5 mg of ipriflavone per kilogram of body weight to rats for forty-five days. The rats were then forced to swim daily until exhaustion with a weight attached to their legs. At the end of the experiment, the ipriflavone-treated animals were able to swim an additional thirty-three minutes (an increase of 39 percent) compared with the controls. A second study found significant (but unspecified) increases in protein synthesis when rats were given 30 mg per kilogram of body weight for three weeks.

Another experiment with rats found that 5 mg of ipriflavone per kilogram of body weight partially suppressed the effect of cortisone, which can be converted into the hormone cortisol. High levels of cortisol can produce a loss of muscle tissue—the opposite of what you want. This mechanism could be partly responsible for the anabolic actions of this nutrient.

A fourth study gave 20 mg of ipriflavone per kilogram of feed to various farm animals for one to four months. It found increases in body weight ranging from 12 percent in guinea pigs to 20 percent in poultry and rabbits. Testing showed that most of the weight gain was meat (muscle) and not fat.

Hopefully, results of this magnitude will be achieved in healthy human subjects. However, the only human study included was on ten hospital patients suffering from pathological thinness. In this case, a dose of 150 mg three times per day produced an average weight increase of 2–3 kg. The length of the study was not provided.

Ipriflavone has been shown to be a very effective treatment for osteoporosis in more than 150 published studies on animals and humans. Because it does not have a direct estrogenic effect, ipriflavone is able to increase bone-mineral density in older women without the problems that estrogen replacement therapy can have, in part by increasing calcium absorption. Ipriflavone reduces osteoporosis in men, too. That's great news, particularly if you're getting on in years.

The Great Unknown

Since most athletes do not suffer from catabolic disorders, they should be able to make greater gains in muscle mass than weakened hospital patients do. Unfortunately, a MEDLINE data search revealed that no studies on the sports benefits of ipriflavone or 5-methyl-7-methoxyisoflavone have been published to date.

Now that the performance benefits of creatine have been established beyond a shadow of a doubt, it would be nice if researchers redirected their efforts to the study of these exciting isoflavones. Only then will we know for sure how effective they are in helping you achieve your sports goals.

CHAPTER 9

RIBOSE

In order to achieve peak performance, your muscle cells need to provide the maximum amount of energy for muscular contraction. They can do this only when they have ample supplies of a chemical compound called ATP, also known as the "energy currency."

In Chapter 2, you learned that creatine is able to increase the resynthesis of ATP, which is the main reason why it is so effective for boosting strength. But under conditions of heavy training, creatine cannot resynthesize ATP fast enough, and energy molecules escape from the muscle cell. If you train again before your body is able to replenish its ATP stores, your strength and energy levels will suffer. Fortunately, studies show that ribose can speed up this restoration process.

A Powerful Simple Sugar

In healthy individuals, the cells of the body contain ample amounts of ATP at rest. These ATP levels are tightly regulated, and there is no way to increase them beyond their maximum concentrations in the cell. Exercise draws upon these supplies for muscle contraction, temporarily reducing the amount available by up to 30 percent.

When oxygen is available in the cell, ATP resynthesis occurs rapidly. However, when there is a temporary shortage of oxygen (anaerobic conditions), the restoration is much slower. After an extremely intense workout, it can take up to four days for ATP levels to return to normal. During this period of time, your strength and performance will be less than optimal due to the lack of energy resources.

The time lag in ATP recovery occurs primarily because there is not enough of a compound called PRPP.

While PRPP can be made from glucose (blood sugar), it is a relatively slow process. Supplemental ribose has been found to quickly increase PRPP levels.

> **PRPP**
>
> PRPP, or 5-phosphoribosyl-1-pyrophosphate, is a naturally occurring metabolite that the body uses to restore levels of ATP after exercise or other physical exertion.

Ribose is a sugar that is found in all living cells. It is the carbohydrate backbone for RNA (ribonucleic acid) and DNA (deoxyribonucleic acid). These nucleic acids contain the information needed for cells to grow, divide, and carry out their normal functions.

Ribose can be converted into an energy molecule known as pyruvate, which allows ATP to be produced in the presence of oxygen. Another function of ribose is the formation of cyclic nucleotides, compounds that help regulate the activity of calcium and other electrolytes (minerals that conduct electricity) in the cell. These nucleotides control the contraction of your heart and skeletal muscles.

While ribose is found in meat and vegetables, you can't get enough from these sources to boost your sports performance. Supplementation is therefore required. "When you consume ribose, it is converted to PRPP through a metabolic pathway that is much quicker than the body's usual slow conversion of glucose," says Tim Ziegenfuss, Ph.D., CSCS. "This increases the supplies of PRPP and dramatically speeds up the restoration of ATP, both by salvaging the breakdown products of ATP metabolism and by helping to produce more ATP from scratch."

Increases in Strength and Performance

A study at Ball State University found that ribose increased power output. Sixteen male athletes took

10 g of ribose or a dextrose placebo two times per day for a three-day loading phase. They did not exercise during these three days. The athletes then performed five days of high-intensity exercise, consisting each day of two bouts of ten-second sprints on a cycle fifteen times in a row with only fifty seconds of rest between each sprint. After the five days, they rested for sixty-five hours but continued to take the ribose or placebo.

The group that took ribose had an increase in average power output of 4.2 percent during the training period, compared with only 0.6 percent for the placebo group. Also, the ribose group felt less fatigued, although the differences were not statistically significant. Even better, the levels of ATP and a similar compound called ADP returned to normal in the ribose group by the end of the sixty-five-hour recovery period, while the placebo group was still 23 percent below pre-exercise levels.

A similar study at Eastern Michigan University found increases in power of up to 10 percent with a dosage of 10 g per day. "This study confirmed that ribose supplementation can improve explosive anaerobic performance during intense training," says Dr. Ziegenfuss, a researcher in the study.

A study with twenty bodybuilders was performed at the University of Delaware. The athletes in this four-week double-blind study took 5 g of ribose or dextrose placebo twice daily. They then performed ten sets of bench presses per day using a three-day-on/one-day-off training cycle. Ribose supplementation increased their one-rep max by 3.2 percent, while the total number of repetitions they could perform rose by 19.6 percent.

Safe and Effective

The athletes who participated in these experiments experienced no side effects, indicating that ribose is a safe supplement. Because it is a simple sugar, this is hardly surprising. However, you should not take more than 20 g per day, as diarrhea and slight decreases in blood glucose levels have been experienced at higher levels.

In fact, a study at the University of Missouri found that the greatest amount of ATP salvaging per gram of ribose occurred at relatively low doses of ribose (up to 5 g). While larger amounts provided greater benefits, the rate of increase declined, suggesting that the body is prepared to handle only so much ribose at a time.

So stick with 5-g doses (a rounded teaspoon), taking it two to four times per day as needed. The best times to take ribose are before and after your workout. This will allow maximum ATP concentrations during the period when your body needs them the most.

As to ribose's effectiveness, this depends on your sport and type of training. Studies have shown that if you work out frequently at a high level of intensity, ribose will provide benefits. Competitive athletes in sports requiring short bursts of maximal work, such as track and field, powerlifting, and bodybuilding, will likely gain the most. However, if you are a weekend athlete or don't do a large volume of intense training, chances are that you won't experience any change from supplementation.

Weekend athletes have five days to recover, so their bodies can restore ATP levels without the help of ribose. And if you aren't hardcore with your training, you probably won't overtax your ATP levels to begin with. But if you frequently exercise with gung-ho intensity, give ribose a try. You may find that it gives you more energy when you work out.

CHAPTER 10

MSM

If you are serious about your training, you have no doubt experienced delayed-onset muscle soreness as well as occasional tendonitis. This muscle soreness is caused by the microcellular damage that can occur from the stresses of your training program. At the microscopic level, the protein filaments that permit muscle contraction lose some of their integrity. Structural damage can also occur in tendons and ligaments.

Some scientists speculate that the lactic acid produced during your sets irritates these injured muscle tissues as well, further increasing the damage. The soreness can begin within hours and often continues for several days after your workout.

MSM supplementation can dramatically reduce this muscle soreness. This white, crystalline powder, technically known as methylsulfonylmethane, is also effective at reducing inflammation, so it can help your "tennis elbow." It inhibits pain impulses along nerve fibers, dilates blood vessels, and increases blood flow, which could reduce the amount of irritating lactic acid inside the muscle cell. Yet, how it actually does these things remains a mystery.

Sulfur Is an Essential Nutrient

It is widely assumed that MSM works because it is a bioavailable source of sulfur. (One-third of the MSM molecule is sulfur by weight.) Sulfur is found in virtually all body tissues, particularly the red blood cells, muscle, skin, hair, and nails. It is also involved in a number of endocrine and neurotransmitter functions.

Sulfur provides raw material for many enzymes and for compounds that protect against toxicity and free-radical damage. Sulfur is the eighth most abundant element in the human body, comprising 0.25 to 0.5 percent of your body weight. Despite these facts, there is no RDA for this vital mineral.

Sulfur is contained in four amino acids: the essential amino acid methionine and the nonessential cysteine, cystine, and taurine. Nutritionists have historically assumed that if you eat enough protein, you will get enough sulfur. However, these are the same people who think that you don't have to take vitamins if you eat right.

Less Soreness Means More Growth

Many athletes report that their soreness drops by as much as 40 percent when they take MSM. Some note that they don't have to use the railing anymore to climb stairs the day after their leg workout! Even better, the apparent decrease in microcellular damage lessens the amount of repair work needed inside the muscle fiber, giving your body more time to build new muscle tissue. Strength levels often increase, permitting more intense workouts. This can lead to greater muscle mass over time, provided of course that you eat right and don't overtrain.

There is little published research on MSM. We do know that it is a metabolite of DMSO, which has been the subject of thousands of studies over the past forty-five years. (About 15 percent of the DMSO molecule metabolizes into MSM in the body.) Logically, if there were a problem with 15 percent of this molecule, we would know it by now.

One unpublished study by Ronald Lawrence, M.D., president of the American Medical Athletic Association and coauthor of *The Miracle of MSM: The Natural Solution for Pain* (Penguin Putnam, 1999), found dramatic improvements in the frequency of connective-tissue injuries with MSM supplementation. The volunteers took 750 mg of MSM or placebo three times per day for four weeks along with standard chiropractic treatment. Even though the subjects in the MSM group were nearly a decade older on average, they experienced significantly less pain and tenderness than the placebo group. They also needed to make 40 percent fewer visits to the chiropractor for assistance.

The Most Effective Dosage

Although your body contains tiny amounts of MSM naturally (about 2 parts per million) from food sources such as milk, vegetables, coffee, and tea, you need to supplement in order to get enough MSM to help your workouts. MSM comes in crystal form, tablets, and capsules. The crystals are much less expensive, but you may find the bitter taste to be intolerable.

If you decide to try crystals, buy a small container. Drink it with juice or other strong-flavored liquid to mask the taste. A level teaspoon of crystals contains 5 g of MSM. Uncoated tablets are easier to take, but swallow quickly. Capsules, of course, do not have an unpleasant taste, but they are more expensive. The decision is yours.

Begin your supplementation at a dose of 1 g per day before your workout. Some athletes who have taken too much too quickly have experienced headaches. It is better to give your body time to adjust to the higher MSM levels. After a week, start taking one dose before your workout and another dose afterward. This will ensure the greatest concentration of MSM during your training session and the postworkout recovery phase. If you still experience soreness, increase each dose to 2 g.

On the days that you don't work out, a single dose is sufficient. Taking it with meals will reduce the likelihood of any gastrointestinal upset. Also, some athletes say that it increases their energy level. If you notice this, don't take it before bedtime, as it may keep you awake. Other benign side effects include smoother skin and stronger nails.

A Few Precautions

MSM is a very safe nutrient. In fact, a study performed at one of the world's leading toxicology centers in Italy found that it is less toxic than table salt. Still, there are big holes in our knowledge of MSM. Therefore, a few precautions are in order.

Clinical observations indicate that MSM has an aspirinlike effect on platelet aggregation, which results in thinner blood. "If you are taking high doses of aspirin or other blood-thinning medications, consult with your physician before taking MSM," says Lawrence. "Also, MSM may interfere with the accuracy of a test for liver damage that measures enzyme levels, so inform your doctor if you are supplementing with this nutrient." In addition, approximately 1 percent of users experience a rash, particularly in warmer climates. If this occurs, reducing the dosage usually eliminates the problem.

More and more athletes are discovering that MSM reduces the muscle soreness and tendonitis that they get from their workouts. This often leads to greater muscle growth and a new enthusiasm at the gym. So give MSM a try. It could eliminate a nutrient deficiency that has been holding back your training progress.

CHAPTER 11

CAFFEINE, EPHEDRINE, AND OTHER DIET AIDS

One of the benefits of participating in sports is that the increased activity level boosts your daily caloric expenditure, helping to reduce body-fat levels. Whether it's lifting weights or playing volleyball on the beach, an active lifestyle helps to reveal your six-pack abs and lean musculature. However, unless you're a marathon runner or triathlete, chances are that you won't burn enough calories to have a physique as defined as you would like.

This reality has led supplement manufacturers to sell a wide variety of diet aids. Most have thermogenic properties. Other products suppress your appetite, boost fat oxidation, or stimulate the release of thyroid hormones. A few of these sup-plements can even improve your sports performance.

Thermogenic
A nutrient that increases your heat production and meta-bolic rate so you burn more calories each day.

Caffeine: An Ancient Stimulant

Caffeine is a traditional part of virtually every culture on Earth. Whether it's consumed in the form of cof-fee, tea, yerba mate, guarana, or cola drinks, nearly everyone has experienced the uplifting sensation of caffeine. Most of us take this stimulating drug daily. Recently, caffeine has been added to a variety of sports drinks, gels, and even bottled waters for its energizing effects.

The caffeine content of a 12-ounce can of cola ranges from 35–46 mg, while black tea has 45–70 mg per 8-ounce cup depending on the strength.

Green tea averages 25 mg per cup. The amount of caffeine in coffee varies even more. A cup of traditional American drip coffee can have as little as 130 mg, while the same amount of espresso has 400 mg.

Bear in mind that coffee, tea, and similar plants contain a variety of natural chemicals in addition to caffeine. Some of these may counteract caffeine's effect, so if your goal is to increase performance or lose body fat, you should consume a supplement with caffeine instead of drinking huge amounts of coffee. It's great for waking up in the morning, but keep it at that.

Caffeine is rapidly absorbed by the body and remains in circulation for more than seven hours. Plasma concentrations reach a peak one hour after it is consumed. It is then slowly metabolized, with a half-life of four to six hours. There is a large variation among individuals in the response to a given caffeine dose. For some, a small amount can cause jitters and sleeplessness, while others can consume large doses without any negative effects. The precise reasons for this variation are unknown, although it is widely recognized that people can build up a tolerance to caffeine.

Another concern with caffeine is its diuretic effect. Clearly, caffeine increases urine output during the first four hours after you consume it. However, the change is not as great as some people believe. Regular-strength coffee increases urine volume by about 10 percent compared with an equal amount of water, while a large dose of caffeine (8.7 mg per kilogram of body weight) was shown to boost output by 30.6 percent. To prevent dehydration, which can reduce performance even if it is so slight that you don't feel thirsty, be sure to drink at least four liters of water per day and more if you participate in prolonged physical activity.

Proven Sports Benefits

Caffeine is a proven performance enhancer. A

wide range of studies has shown that it increases endurance, speed, and power in a variety of sports. There is also evidence that caffeine boosts strength. Some of these studies used a standard 250-mg dose, which was administered to all subjects regardless of weight. Other studies gave the participants a fixed amount per kilogram of body weight. This latter procedure is much more precise, because caffeine makes its way into—and has effects in—many different body tissues.

A study by researchers at RMIT University in Australia and the University of Otago in New Zealand compared the effects of 6 mg/kg and 9 mg/kg of caffeine on performance during a 2,000-meter rowing exercise. Eight competitive oarsmen completed the rowing tests on different days. Compared with the results without caffeine, there was an average reduction in rowing time of 1.2 percent and an increase in mean power of 2.7 percent. There was no significant difference between the two dosage levels, suggesting that more is not always better with caffeine.

Caffeine also helps swimmers. A study published in the *Canadian Journal of Applied Physiology* found significant reductions in swim times. Time to completion for the 500-meter race dropped by seven seconds when 6 mg/kg of caffeine was consumed, while the improvement for the 1,500-meter race was twenty-three seconds. Similar benefits have been noted in studies with cyclists. A study involving soldiers at training camp even showed that it moderately increased the time to exhaustion during intense drills.

Caffeine has also been shown to boost strength levels. A study at York University in Toronto found that 5 mg/kg increased maximum lifting weight by 3.5 percent, while the time to fatigue for exercise performed at 50 percent of the one-rep max rose by 26 percent. This suggests that caffeine has a localized effect within the muscle fibers.

These and other studies show that caffeine can improve sports performance at doses between 3 and 6 mg/kg. This is important because caffeine use is limited at the Olympics and other major sports events. You may have been under the impression that caffeine was prohibited at the Olympics, but this is an overstatement.

The International Olympic Committee (IOC) has set a limit of 12 mcg of caffeine per milliliter of urine. Yet most people would have to take an acute dose of 9 mg/kg to get close to 12 mcg per milliliter. Clearly, you can get a performance benefit from caffeine and still pass your IOC drug test. Remember, however, that not everyone gets the same urinary concentration from a given dose of caffeine. For unknown reasons, some athletes excrete more than others do. Most people are safe at 6 mg/kg, but if you are competing at the elite level, you might want to test your levels beforehand to be sure.

Athletes are sometimes told that the sports benefits of caffeine will occur only if they avoid regular use of caffeine and caffeinated beverages. Research has shown this to be false, however. Comparative studies have revealed no difference in performance between regular users and abstainers. (The drug clears your system within forty-eight hours.) So if you want a cup of Joe in the morning, go right ahead.

How Caffeine Works

There are a number of theories about how caffeine improves performance. Traditionally, it was felt that caffeine works by increasing free fatty-acid levels. This provides an additional source of fuel that "spares" the glycogen stores. While it is true that some (but not all) studies show a rise in fatty acids, lactate levels also go up, indicating an increase in the use of blood glucose and glycogen for fuel. So little sparing may actually be going on.

Besides, the availability of substrates such as fat and carbohydrate is rarely a limit on performance for exercise lasting less than sixty minutes. If you are a marathon runner or triathlete, caffeine may actually help you to maintain your performance longer by increasing the time before you use up your glycogen stores (also called "hitting the wall"). But it is unlikely that this mechanism explains the benefits for athletes who do short-term, intense exercise, such as weightlifters and sprinters.

Recent studies suggest that an important mechanism of action for caffeine is increasing adrenaline levels.

Caffeine has also been shown to stimulate uptake of potassium into muscle cells. Since the loss of potassium is partly responsible for muscle fatigue, this mechanism results in prolonged activation in the motor units of the muscle fibers and greater force production. Caffeine changes the ionic balance within muscle tissue, as well.

Adrenaline

Adrenaline is a hormone released during stressful situations. Often called the "fight or flight" hormone, it binds to the receptors in many tissues and increases alertness, allowing athletes to function at a higher performance level.

There is no question that caffeine is an important ergogenic aid. But can it help you to lose body fat? Don't count on it. Several studies have looked at caffeine doses ranging from 100–600 mg per day. While caffeine had a mild thermogenic effect and slightly increased fat burning, the differences were not statistically significant compared with the placebo. The increased adrenaline level may reduce your appetite somewhat, but that's about all. Yet, when you combine caffeine with ephedrine, it's a different story.

Ephedrine Boosts Performance

Ephedrine is a natural chemical found in the *Ephedra sinica* plant, from which it gets its name. Also known as ma huang, this plant has a long history of usage in Asian countries for the treatment of asthma and other bronchial conditions. A related chemical, pseudoephedrine, is also found in the plant and is an ingredient in many cold and flu remedies.

Ephedrine is a stimulant that works on the receptors in the central nervous system. It has been shown to increase the level of dopamine, which is a precursor to both epinephrine and norepinephrine, both vital neurotransmitters. Dopamine is also an important neurotransmitter around the hypothalamus, an area of the brain that is important for body arousal. Unlike caffeine, which exerts many of its benefits in muscle tissue, ephedrine appears to work primarily on the central nervous system.

Several studies have looked at ephedrine's role in improving sports performance. It appears that significant gains can be achieved only when you take at least 1 mg per kilogram of body weight. Less than that is not effective.

For example, a study at Victoria Hospital and the University of Western Ontario gave 24 mg of ephedrine to twenty-one young males who then performed an extensive battery of tests designed to measure everything from muscle strength, endurance, and power to lung function, VO_{2max}, and recovery time. About the only thing that ephedrine did was increase the average heart rate. A similar study with 120 mg of pseudoephedrine showed no benefit during one hour of high-intensity exercise, although it should be noted the pseudoephedrine is only a third as strong as ephedrine.

On the other hand, studies at the Defense and Civil Institute of Environmental Medicine in Toronto showed positive results. Unlike the debate about doping in athletic events, no one has a problem with giving ephedrine to soldiers if it can increase their fighting potential. When 1 mg/kg was given to sixteen healthy males, there was a significant increase in power output during the first fifteen seconds of a thirty-second test that measures anaerobic power. Another study by this institute found that the same amount of ephedrine increased the time to exhaustion on a set of military drills by 19 percent.

The King of Thermogenics

Ephedrine is an effective fat burner on its own. Renowned weight-loss expert Arne Astrup, M.D., and his associates performed a study at the University of Copenhagen and two Danish hospitals. Five young females were given 20 mg of ephedrine three times per day one hour before meals and were told to continue eating normally. Even though there was no dieting involved, the women lost an average of 2.5 kilograms of body weight after four weeks and 5.5 kilograms after twelve weeks. They also held on to their lean muscle, while their body-fat percentage dropped by 3.5 percent after four weeks and 5.2 percent after twelve weeks. Two months after the experiment stopped, they had only gained back 0.5 kilograms. The only side effect was a mild rise in blood pressure at the start of the experiment.

When ephedrine is combined with caffeine, the effects are even greater. This combination has been extensively studied, but space limitations do not allow a detailed listing of the many studies that have showed benefits. All of this research, however, supports the effectiveness of the E/C stack (combination of ephedrine and caffeine) and demonstrates the moderate level of side effects that occur when you take specific dosages.

Two studies by the same Danish researchers indicate the extent of the benefits. In both studies, the participants took a supplement with 20 mg of ephedrine and 200 mg of caffeine three times per day. They also followed a low-calorie diet. In the first study, the test subjects lost 16.2 percent of their body weight in twenty-four weeks, significantly more than the 13.4 percent loss by the placebo group. The second study confirmed that most of this loss was body fat. In that eight-week study, the E/C group lost 10.1 kg, compared with only 8.4 kg with the placebo. But the E/C group lost twice as much fat (9.0 kg versus 4.5 kg) and much less fat-free mass (1.1 kg versus 3.9 kg). Only mild side effects, such as upset stomach and jitteriness, were reported in some individuals.

While the mechanisms are still not known, it is thought that caffeine has a "permissive" action on ephedrine, lowering the amount needed to achieve its physiological effects. In other words, caffeine potentiates ephedrine's effect. The E/C studies that showed the greatest benefits used a 10:1 ratio of caffeine to ephedrine, so be sure to use a supplement that contains this ratio.

Some products contain natural plant extracts as the sources for these nutrients. Guarana, for example, is a source of caffeine. If the product uses an extract, look for the amount of the active ingredient on the label. It is the active ingredients that must be in a 10:1 ratio—not the amount of extract, which can come in varying concentrations.

Some thermogenic supplements add aspirin or willow-bark extract to the basic E/C combination. (Willow bark is a natural source of salicin, which is similar to the acetylsalicylic acid in aspirin.) These ingredients are said to further increase the effects of the E/C stack by helping to raise the body's set point for temperature regulation and keeping the body from reregulating itself. This would boost the basal metabolic rate and help to burn more body fat. However, this may not always be the case.

"While a study with obese mice showed that aspirin contributed to energy expenditure, one human study showed no improvement compared to ephedrine and caffeine alone, and another found significant benefits only in obese individuals," notes Will Brink, author of the e-book *Diet Supplements Revealed* (www.aboutsupplements.com). "So aspirin may not provide a benefit in athletes. Studies still need to be performed in these individuals."

A number of studies have been published in

which entire over-the-counter products with caffeine, ephedrine, aspirin or willow bark, and other ingredients were tested and found to be effective compared with a placebo. However, since additional substances were involved, the role of the aspirin or willow bark cannot be established. Only time will tell the precise role of salicin or acetylsalicylic acid in athletes.

Be Aware of Possible Side Effects

The studies on ephedrine and caffeine reported very few side effects with the use of these stimulants in healthy subjects. There were occasional reports of headaches, irritability, anxiety, and tremors. These effects were most frequent during the first week or two of supplementation, after which the study participants seemed to get accustomed to the stimulation.

However, there is a wide variability in how an individual responds to these plant chemicals. Some people, for example, can drink coffee all day and fall asleep easily, while others wind up staring at the ceiling if they have coffee for lunch. Start out with a half-dose to see how you respond to these strong stimulants, and never exceed the recommended dosage.

Some studies have reported a mild increase in heart rate or blood pressure, especially at the start of the study. As a result, if you have high blood pressure, you should not take these stimulants. If your blood pressure is high-normal, bear in mind that caffeine and ephedrine could push you into the high range. If you are in this category, you should ideally measure your blood pressure before you begin supplementation and then again a month later to see if any change has taken place.

Also, do not use caffeine or ephedrine if you are pregnant or breast-feeding, elderly, under age eighteen, or chronically ill. Talk to your doctor before using these stimulants if you are taking any prescription or over-the-counter medication, including but not limited to antidepressants, stimulants, allergy medications, and drugs for cardio-vascular conditions.

Skip your afternoon dose if you have trouble sleeping, and discontinue use entirely if you feel any dizziness, nausea, anxiety, headaches, or heart palpitations. You can still lose weight through a sensible diet and exercise regimen. It will take a while longer, but that's better than worsening a medical condition.

More Thermogenic Options

Caffeine is found in a variety of plants, and extracts of these plants are sometimes included in thermogenic supplements. Guarana (*Paullinia cupana*) is a shrub that is native to Brazil. It contains caffeine and traces of related alkaloids, as do kola nut, yerba mate, and various teas. These extracts may be added to thermogenic products instead of, or in addition to, the usual caffeine from coffee.

While these herbs and plants may be advertised as "natural" alternatives to the caffeine in coffee, don't be misled. Coffee is also a natural plant grown in mountainous regions around the world. Quite simply, caffeine is caffeine. Your body neither knows nor cares what plant it came from. However, because the caffeine content of these plants varies, be sure to check for the amount of caffeine in the extract. That is what should be in the 10:1 ratio with ephedrine.

Citrus aurantium, also called bitter orange, contains synephrine, a compound that is similar to ephedrine. Although not as strong as ephedrine, it increases metabolic activity and boosts thermo-genesis. It does not suppress appetite, however. Because *Citrus aurantium* produces fewer side effects, it is a good choice if you find that you are sensitive to ephedrine.

Sida cordifolia is another source of ephedrine, but it is not found in high concentrations in the plant. Be sure to check the strength of the *Sida cordifolia* extract you are considering using. Norephedrine, another cousin to ephedrine, has a stimulating effect similar to these two compounds. These products are normally part of a combination weight-loss product and are rarely sold separately.

Carnitine and HCA Boost Fat Oxidation

You can also lose body fat by increasing the rate at which you oxidize the fats, or lipids, in your bloodstream. Hydroxycitric acid (HCA) and carnitine have been shown to assist in this process. The enzyme that regulates fatty-acid oxidation is carnitine palmitoyl transferase-1 (CPT-1). It transports fat into the mitochondria (energy factory) of the cell for oxidation. When you supplement with carnitine, you increase the supply of the main raw material needed to activate CPT-1, which can boost the amount of fat oxidation that takes place. Take 1–3 g of carnitine per day to maximize this process.

HCA is an acid that comes from the rind of *Garcinia cambogia.* This grapefruit-sized fruit, also known as Malabar tamarind, has been used as a condiment for thousands of years in India. Scientists now know that HCA inhibits the action of citrate lyase, an enzyme that reduces the level of lipid oxidation in the body. By putting the handcuffs on citrate lyase, you increase the body's propensity to burn fats while decreasing the utilization of carbohydrates. This has the effect of keeping more carbs in the liver, which is where your hunger receptors are located. End result: less hunger.

HCA works best in combination with carnitine, since this allows you to alter the oxidation equation on both sides. Take 2–6 g of HCA per day at the same time you take your carnitine. Some diet supplements contain both nutrients.

Guggulsterones and Thyroid Boosters

The thyroid gland plays a pivotal role in regulating your metabolism. It releases hormones that increase

the rate at which your cells release energy from carbohydrates, while promoting protein synthesis and
the utilization of fatty acids. If your thyroid does not
release as many of these hormones as the average
person, you are said to have a "slow metabolism."
On the other hand, if the thyroid gland releases too
much of these hormones, you could end up with a
catabolic condition known as muscle wasting.

Guggulsterones are the active ingredients in
guggul lipids, which are fatty substances that are
extracted from the herb *Commiphora mukul.* For
centuries, practitioners of the traditional Ayurvedic
system of medicine have recommended this Indian
plant for weight loss. It appears to promote the production of thyroid hormones, helping to counteract
the usual slowing of the metabolic rate during a
diet. While there is little Western research on this
nutrient, it has been shown to reduce cholesterol
levels by lowering the amount of LDL (the "bad"
cholesterol), so you may get a double benefit.

Coleus forskohili is another thyroid booster.
The active ingredient in the plant, called forskolin,
has been shown to increase the efficiency of T3, an
important thyroid hormone. "Coleus enhances T3
efficiency by increasing the level of cyclic AMP,
which is a gatekeeper for energy regulation," says
Dallas Clouatre, Ph.D., author of *Anti-Fat Nutrients*
(Pax, 1997). "This results in a greater metabolic
expenditure and will help to reduce body-fat levels as long as your diet and exercise regimens are
appropriate."

Other Diet Supplements

A number of other products are sold as weight-loss
enhancers. One is alpha lipoic acid (ALA). In people
with diabetes, ALA increases insulin sensitivity,
which is the body's ability to respond to a rise in
blood glucose. The theory is that higher insulin levels will shunt more of the glucose into the muscle
cells, so it won't be stored as body fat. While this

may be true, there is no published evidence to date that it occurs in healthy athletes. ALA is a strong antioxidant, however.

Chromium is a mineral that helps insulin bind to its receptor sites. It is also involved in the metabolism of glucose for energy. A deficiency of chromium can lead to increased fat storage, fatigue, sugar cravings, and mood swings, all of which are counterproductive to your weight-loss goals. The average American diet does not provide enough chromium for a sedentary person, much less an athlete. For this reason, you should supplement with 200 mcg of chromium picolinate per day and eat plenty of chromium-rich whole-grain cereals.

Tyrosine is an amino acid that plays an important role in human metabolism. It is the precursor to stimulatory neurotransmitters such as epinephrine, norepinephrine, dopamine, and some of the thyroid hormones. While there is no published evidence that tyrosine works on its own as a weight-loss agent, several studies have shown that it increases the benefits of caffeine/ephedrine products, in part by helping to curb appetite. Tyrosine also appears to reduce stress and fatigue, so you can more easily stick to your diet. If your weight-loss supplement does not include tyrosine, try taking 500 mg of tyrosine along with it. You may find that this amino acid enhances its effectiveness.

With the wide variety of weight-loss products available, it's easy to get confused. Most, however, contain various combinations of the nutrients mentioned in this chapter. Because individual sensitivities vary, always start with a small dose and work your way up. You've wanted to lose weight for some time now—another week or two won't make a big difference. And be sure to control your food intake and exercise regularly. Diet supplements are a lot more effective when you give them a helping hand!

CHAPTER 12

SPORTS DRINKS

Not that long ago, the category of sports drinks had one entry: Gatorade. Originally developed for the Gators football team at the University of Florida, Gatorade became a household word with the once-revolutionary concept that water is not the best thing to drink during exercise.

When studies confirmed that drinks with electrolytes and simple carbohydrates improved sports performance, a new market segment was born. It has since grown to a billion-dollar industry with a large number of entries and an ever-expanding variety of flavors. While it is not possible in this short book to review them all, this chapter will discuss the five main types of sports drinks available for consumers. Depending on your sport and recovery goals, all of these drinks may be appropriate for you at one time or another.

Low-Carb Drinks Reduce Fatigue

The earliest sports drinks were all low-carb drinks. These Gatorade competitors are designed to be consumed before and during exercise. They provide a relatively low amount of simple carbs that helps to maintain your blood-sugar levels during exercise. This carbohydrate usually comes from sucrose, glucose, glucose polymers, fructose, or high-fructose corn syrup.

These drinks are around 6 to 8 percent carbs, so they are predominantly water. This makes them valuable sources of fluids to replace the water lost through perspiration and breathing. The low carb level also maximizes fluid absorption while minimizing stomach upset during exercise.

Low-carb drinks also contain the electrolytes sodium and potassium. This helps to restore the appropriate levels of these minerals, which are lost during training. Another advantage of sodium is that it increases thirst, encouraging the appropriate consumption of fluids to keep your body fully hydrated.

The drinks are equally beneficial for strength and endurance athletes, who need to maintain their energy levels during exercise. Since most forms of sustained exercise primarily use glucose and glycogen for energy, providing small amounts of carbs can help to prevent a loss of training intensity.

Don't go overboard drinking low-carb drinks. They are intended to be sipped in small amounts, not guzzled a bottle at a time. If you overdo it, you could experience gastric distress. Too many carbs right before or during exercise also reduces the beneficial hormonal responses to exercise. In moderation, however, low-carb drinks can reduce fatigue and promote maximal performance.

High-Carb Drinks Promote Glycogen Resynthesis

High-carb drinks contain two to four times as many carbs as the low-carb versions. They should not be used during exercise, because they can upset your stomach if consumed too quickly and can reduce desirable elevations in testosterone and growth hormone. However, after exercise they provide a convenient way to get the carbs you need right after your workout to maximize glycogen resynthesis.

Studies have shown that your first meal after a workout should be an easily digestible meal such as a sports drink or meal-replacement drink. These drinks are assimilated quicker than a meal from whole food, allowing you to start the rebuilding process as soon as possible. This can help to minimize muscle breakdown as well.

One of the advantages of high-carb drinks is that they can be mixed with creatine to form an impromptu creatine-transport drink. They can also be used to increase total calorie count if you are on a weight-gain diet. Some brands contain electrolytes, vitamin C, and chromium and other minerals, while others are pure carb beverages.

High-carb drinks are made from the same simple sugars used for the low-carb drinks, with possibly some maltodextrin or other complex carbohydrate added. This makes them beneficial after a workout when your primary objective is rebuilding your glycogen stores. However, you shouldn't live on simple sugars. Use these drinks as postworkout beverages, and eat mainly complex carbohydrates the rest of the day.

Protein Drinks Provide Essential Amino Acids

Protein drinks are an easy way to get the high-quality protein you need to recover and build muscle. These beverages can be put in a gym bag or briefcase, allowing you to get essential amino acids right after your workout or when you are on the run and don't have access to a blender to mix a regular protein shake.

These drinks are usually made from whey protein, although some contain casein and/or soy as well. The amount of protein varies with the size of the container, although most provide between 20 and 45 g. Some drinks have additional ingredients, ranging from vitamins and minerals to nutrients that may increase uptake and delivery of amino acids to the muscle cells. Others provide added glutamine or branched-chain amino acids. Most have very little carbs and fat.

Many of the products in this category are ready-to-drink beverages, but some of them come in powdered form. While these powder drinks have the disadvantage that you need to fill the bottles with cold water, they do provide a mess-free, pre-measured dose of protein powder. They are also much lighter than the liquid drinks. This could be an advantage depending on the number that you are carrying.

Recovery Drinks Combine Carbs and Protein

Recovery drinks were originally designed as post-workout beverages, but new research at the University of Texas shows that they can also boost performance when taken during exercise. These drinks usually contain 10–15 g of protein and 15–35 g of carbs with little or no fat. A few have higher carb levels. Since your body needs both carbs and protein to maximize recovery, these combination drinks can be very beneficial.

"There is some evidence that protein helps the uptake of carbs, even during exercise," notes Edmund Burke, Ph.D., author of *Optimal Muscle Recovery* (Avery Publishing, 1999). "Research has shown that a sports drink with carbs and protein improves the fuel efficiency and recovery of muscle even better than a drink that only has carbohydrates."

The study at the University of Texas used a 4:1 ratio of carbs to protein. Scientists found that this amount of protein provided essential amino acids without negatively impacting fluid and car-bohydrate replenishment. Too much protein, the researchers warned, could reduce these benefits, so you should try to maintain this ratio during the two hours after your workout. This would require the intake of more carbs than the amount contained in most recovery drinks.

Even with the macronutrients in these drinks, they have substantial amounts of water. This makes it easier to rehydrate after a workout. Also, since intense training decreases appetite, these drinks offer a convenient and flavorful way to get the nutrients you need to recover and increase your strength.

Fat-Burner Drinks Help You Lose Weight

These drinks contain no protein and virtually no carbs. What they do have are fat-burning nutrients such as ephedra, caffeine, guarana, white willow bark, hydroxycitric acid, and carnitine. While these supplements are also available in capsule form, consuming them in a drink gives you a flavorful beverage with water (which is especially important while you are dieting).

All of these nutrients are stable in water, so there is no loss of potency as occurs with creatine. You pay more for the nutrients when they are in sports drinks instead of pills, but there is a convenience factor involved as well as a taste advantage.

If you are sensitive to stimulants or only want to take a small amount of them, consuming a drink may give you all of the assistance you need to shed unwanted pounds. However, because fat-burners can cause side effects in some individuals, please read Chapter 11 before taking these nutrients.

CONCLUSION

Every athlete wants to reach his or her goal as soon as possible. Nowadays, that means you have to eat right, train hard, and take a variety of sports nutrients to ensure your progress. These supplements can increase your strength and muscle size, enhance endurance, and keep your immune system strong, making them essential tools in your training regimen.

This guide has given you a good understanding of the leading sports nutrients in the marketplace. Armed with this knowledge, you can now make the best purchases for your own needs. You can tailor your supplement program to match your sport and intensity level, while keeping your expenses down to a minimum.

At the same time, never loose track of the fact that sports excellence does not come in a bottle. Sports nutrients are meant to supplement a healthy diet with plenty of protein, carbs, and healthy fats. They cannot make up for poor workouts, either, so don't use them as a crutch. Stick to a focused exercise regimen that provides plenty of training stimuli along with sufficient time for rest and recuperation.

When you give it your all at the gym or on the playing field, you'll find that these valuable nutrients will return the favor by giving you the maximum benefits they have to offer. Best of luck on your sports progress!

SELECTED
REFERENCES

Astrup, A, Lundsgaard, C, Madsen, J, et al. Enhanced thermogenic responsiveness during chronic ephedrine treatment in man. *The American Journal of Clinical Nutrition*, 1985; 42:83–94.

Bucci, L. Selected herbals and human exercise performance. *American Journal of Clinical Nutrition*, 2000; 72(suppl):624S–636S.

Burke, E. *Optimal Muscle Recovery*. Garden City Park, NY: Avery Publishing Group, 1999.

Clarkson, P and Haymes, E. Trace mineral requirements for athletes. *International Journal of Sport Nutrition*, 1994; 4:104–119.

Dinan, L. Phytoecdysteroids: Biological aspects. *Phytochemistry*, 2001; 57:325–339.

Fahey, T and Pearl M. The hormonal and perceptive effects of phosphatidylserine administration during two weeks of resistive exercise-induced overtraining. *Biology of Sport*, 1998; 15:135–143.

Graham, T. Caffeine and exercise: metabolism, endurance and performance. *Sports Medicine*, 2001; 31(11):785–807.

Jacob, S., Lawrence, R., and Zucker, M. *The Miracle of MSM: The Natural Solution for Pain*. New York: Penguin Putnam, 1999.

Lemon, P. Do athletes need more dietary protein and amino acids? *International Journal of Sport Nutrition*, 1995; 5:S39–S61.

Sahelian, R, and Tuttle, D. *Creatine: Nature's Muscle Builder.* Garden City Park, NY: Avery Publishing Group, 1999.

Van Der Beek, E. Vitamin supplementation and physical exercise performance. *Journal of Sports Sciences,* 1991; 9:77–89.

Welbourne, T. Increased plasma bicarbonate and growth hormone after an oral glutamine load. *American Journal of Clinical Nutrition,* 1995; 61: 1058–1061

Witter, J., Gallagher, P., Williamson, D., et al. Effects of ribose supplementation on performance during repeated high-intensity cycle sprints. Abstract presented at the Midwest Regional Chapter of the American College of Sports Medicine, October 2000.

OTHER BOOKS
AND RESOURCES

Burke, E. *Optimal Muscle Recovery.* Garden City Park, NY: Avery Publishing Group, 1999.

Challem, J., and Brown, L. *User's Guide to Vitamins and Minerals,* North Bergen, New Jersey: Basic Health Publications, 2002.

Di Pasquale, M. *Amino Acids and Proteins and the Athlete: An Anabolic Edge.* [CITY:] CRC Press, 1997.

Sahelian, R., and Tuttle, D. *Creatine: Nature's Muscle Builder.* Garden City Park, NY: Avery Publishing Group, 1997.

Tuttle, D. *50 Ways to Build Muscle Fast.* Garden City Park, NY: Avery Publishing Group, 1999.

Wilmore, J., and Costill, D. *Physiology of Sport and Exercise.* Champaign, Illinois: Human Kinetics, 1999.

GreatLife Magazine
Consumer magazine with articles on vitamins, minerals, herbs, and foods.
Available for free at many health and natural food stores.

Let's Live Magazine
Consumer magazine with emphasis on the health benefits of vitamins, minerals, and herbs.
Customer service:
1-800-676-4333
P.O. Box 74908
Los Angeles, CA 90004
Subscriptions: 12 issues per year, $19.95 in the U.S.; $31.95 outside the U.S.

Physical Magazine

Magazine oriented to body builders and other serious athletes.

Customer service:

1-800-676-4333

P.O. Box 74908

Los Angeles, CA 90004

Subscriptions: 12 issues per year, $19.95 in the U.S.; $31.95 outside the U.S.

The Nutrition Reporter™ newsletter

Monthly newsletter that summarizes recent medical research on vitamins, minerals, and herbs.

Customer service:

P.O. Box 30246

Tucson, AZ 85751-0246

e-mail: jack@thenutritionreporter.com

www.nutritionreporter.com

Subscriptions: $26 per year (12 issues) in the U.S.; $32 U.S. or $48 CNC for Canada; $38 for other countries

INDEX

Actin, 4
Adaptogen, 37
Adenosine diphosphate (ADP), 12, 61
Adenosine triphosphate (ATP), 11–12, 59–62
Adrenaline, 71
Aerobic pathway, 12–13
Alanine, 4
Alpha-lipoic acid (ALA), 18, 78–79
Amino acids, 3–4, 6, 13, 17, 24–25, 27–29, 39–40, 63–64, 82–83
Ammonia, 28
Angelica sinensis, 43
Anti-Fat Nutrients, 78
Antioxidant glutathione, 7
Antioxidants, 32
Arginine, 4, 6, 7, 13, 18, 28
Asparagine, 4
Aspartic acid, 4
Aspirin, 74–75
Astragalus, 42, 48–50
Astrup, Arne, 73
Athletes, 3–10, 11–22, 23–30, 31–36, 37–41, 42–54, 55–58, 59–62, 63–66, 67–79, 80–85
Ayurvedic medicine, 78

Beer, 55–56
Bioavailabilty, 7, 33
Biochanin A, 55
Biotin, 31
Bitter orange, 76
Bloating, 16
Blood cells, 3, 26, 35
Blood pressure, 75
Bones, 35
Brain cells, 3
Brink, Will, 74
Burke, Edmund, 83

Caffeine, 67–71, 75–76
Calcium, 32, 34, 35–36
Canadian Journal of Applied Physiology, 69
Carbohydrates, 5, 8, 9, 10
  daily requirements, 10
Carnitine, 77
Casein, 6–7, 9
China, 42

Chlorine, 33
Cholesterol, *See* LDL.
Chromium, 33, 79
Chromium picolinate, 79
Citrus aurantium, 76
Clouatre, Dallas, 78
Cobalt, 33
Codonopsis pilosula, 43
Coenzymes, 32
Colds, 26
Coleus forskohlii, 78
Commiphora mukul, 78
Copper, 33
Cortisol, 51–53
CPT-1, 77
Creapure, 13
Creatine, 11–22, 27, 59, 82
  dosages, 14–15, 20–21
Creatine candy, 11
Creatine citrate, 11, 16–17, 18, 19
  dosages, 16
Creatine, effervescent, 11, 18–19
Creatine, free, 11
Creatine, liquid, 11, 19–20
Creatine monohydrate, 11, 14, 16–17, 18, 19
Creatine phosphate, 11
Creatine-transport drinks, 11, 17–18
Creatine: Nature's Muscle Builder, 14
Creatinine, 14, 19
Cyclic nucleotides, 60
Cysteine, 4

d-alpha tocopherol. *See* Vitamin E.
Dean, Joan, 20
Deoxyribonucleic acid (DNA), 60
Diabetes, 18, 78, 79
Diet, 3–10
Diet Supplements Revealed, 74
Diuretics, 68
dl-alpha tocopherol. *See* Vitamin E.
DMSO, 64
Dopamine, 72
D-pinitol, 18

Ecdysone, 39
Ecdysteroids, 37–41

Ecdysterone, 37–41
Egg albumin, 9
Egg powders, 6
*Eksperimentalnaia I Klinicheskaia
    Farmakologiia*, 41
Electrolytes, 80–84
Eleutheroccus senticosus, 42, 46
Energy, 43
Energy pathways, 11–12
Enzymes, 36, 55, 77
Ephedrine, 71–77
Ethnopharmacology, 44

Fahey, Thomas, 51–53
Fat, 5, 8, 9, 10
Fat blockers, 9
Fat burner drinks, 84
Fat burners, 9, 73–79, 84
Federal Drug Administration, 30
Fiber, 10
5-methyl-7-methoxyisoflavone,
    56
5-phosphoribosyl-1-
    pyrophosphate, 60
Flavones, 55
Fluorine, 33
Folic acid, 31. *See also* Vitamin
    B complex.
Free radicals, 32, 34
Fu Zheng therapy, 48

Garcinia cambogia, 77
Gatorade, 80
Ginseng, 42–50
    forms, 47
    root extract, 46
    synergy with astragalus, 49–50
    types, 42–44
Ginsenosides, 47
GH. *See* Growth hormone.
Glehnia littoralis, 43
Glucose, 8
Glutamic acid, 4
Glutamine, 4, 6, 7, 24–27
Glycine, 4, 13
Glycogen, 8
Glycogen resynthesis, 81–82
Glycolysis, 12
Growth factors, 9
Growth hormone, 4, 23–30
Guarana, 74, 76
Guggulsterones, 77–78

Half-life, 39
HCA, 77
Herbs, 37–41, 42–50, 76
    adaptogenic, 37
Herpes simplex, 28

High-carb drinks, 81–82
Histidine, 4
Homeopathy, 29–30
Hormones, 4, 51, 55
Hydroxycitric acid, 77

Immune system, 9, 24–26, 41, 48
Insulin, 4, 18, 78, 79
*International Clinical Nutrition
    Review*, 45
Iodine, 33
Ion-exchange, 7
Ipriflavone, 55, 57–58
Iron, 33
Isoleucine, 4

Japanese Journal of Hygiene, 48

Karolinska Institute, 15
Kilogram, 5

Lactic acid, 12, 24, 27, 63
Lactose, 6–7
Lawrence, Ronald, 64, 66
LDL, 41, 78
L-dopa, 29
Lead, 33
Lemon, Peter, 4
Leucine, 4
*Leuzea carthamoides. See
    Rhaponticum carthamoides.*
Life Extension, 29
Low-carb drinks, 80–81
Low-density lipoprotein.
    See LDL.
Lysine, 4, 27, 28

Ma huang. *See* Ephedrine.
Magnesium, 33, 34, 36
Malabar tamarind, 77
Manganese, 33
Meal frequency, 8
Meal-replacement powders
    (MRPs), 3, 6–10
Methionine, 4, 6, 13
Methoxyisoflavone, 49, 55–56, 58
Methylsufonylmethane, 63–66
Microfiltration, 7
Micronutrients, 31
Milk powders, 6
Minerals, 9, 31–36
*Miracle of MSM: The Natural
    Solution for Pain*, 64
Molybdenum, 33
MSM, 63–66
Muscle cells, 3, 24–25
Muscle growth, 5, 9, 10, 14,
    23–30, 31–36, 63–66

Muscle fiber, 11
Myosin, 4

Nerve cells, 52, 72
Nervous system, 72
Neurotransmitters, 29, 72, 79
Niacin. *See* Vitamin B$_3$.
Nickel, 33
Nitric oxide, 27
Nitrogen balance, 4–5, 24
Norephedrine, 77
Nucleic acids, 60
Nutrients, 8

Optimal Muscle Recovery, 83
Orange juice, 19
Osteoporosis, 56, 57

Panax ginseng, 42–49
Panax japonica, 43
Panax quinquefolius, 42, 45–46,
    49
Panax pseudoginseng, 43
Pantothenic acid, 31
Pearson, Durk, 29
Peptides, bioactive, 9
Pfaffia paniculata, 38
Phenylalanine, 4, 7
Phosphatidylserine, 51–54
Phosphorus, 32
Phylloquinone. *See* Vitamin K.
Polysaccharides, 47
Potassium, 33, 71
Pregnancy, 75
Proline, 4
Protein, 3–10
Protein drinks, 82–83
Protein powders, 3, 6–8, 10
PRPP, 60
Pseudoephedrine, 71
Pseudostellaria heterophylla,
    43
Pyruvate, 60

Qi, 43, 45

Recovery drinks, 83
Rhaponticum carthamoides,
    38–39, 40, 46
Ribonucleic acid, 60
Ribose, 59–62
Ribosomes, 39–40
Rogers, Michael, 50

Sahelian, Ray, 14
Schizophrenia, 28
Secretagogues, 23–30
Selenium, 33

Semen, 27
Serine, 4
Shaw, Sandy, 29
Sida cordifolia, 76
Silicon, 33
Sodium, 33
Somatostatin, 29
Soviet Union, 37
Soy isolate, 6
Soy powders, 6
Spinach, 39
Sports drinks, 80–84
Standardized Profile of Mood
    States, 50
Sugar, 60
Sulfur, 32, 63
Sweetners, natural, 19
Synephrine, 76

Teeth, 35
Tendonitis, 64–66
Thermogenics, 67, 73–76
Thiamine. *See* Vitamin B$_1$.
Threonine, 4
Thyroid, 77–78
Thyroid boosters, 77–78
Tin, 33
Tryptophan, 4
T-3, 78
20-hydroxyecdysone, 38–41
    studies on, 40
Tyrosine, 29, 79

Valine, 4
Vegetables, 34
Vitamin A, 31, 32
Vitamin B Complex, 32
Vitamin B$_1$, 31,
Vitamin B$_2$, 31
Vitamin B$_3$, 31
Vitamin B$_6$, 31
Vitamin B$_{12}$, 31
Vitamin C, 31, 32, 34
Vitamin D, 31, 32
Vitamin E, 31, 32, 33, 34
Vitamin K, 31, 32
Vitamins, 9, 31–36
VO$_{2max}$, 43, 45, 46

Wei qi, 48
Weight loss, 67–79
Welbourne, Tomas, 25
Whey, 6–7, 9, 82
Willow bark, 74–75
Wound healing, 27

Ziegenfuss, Tim, 60, 61
Zinc, 33